Bob Barefoot On Vitamin-D

"The Cancer Inhibitor"

By

Robert R. Barefoot

© Copyright 2005
Robert R. Barefoot
Web Site "www.cureamerica.net"

D0011895

Who is usually deficient in Vitamin-D ?

http://my.webmd.com/content/article/78/95751.htm In the latest study, Gregory A. Plotnikoff, MD, of the University of Minnesota Medical School stated *that all of the African Americans, East Africans, Hispanics, and Native Americans who participated in the study were vitamin-D deficient,* as were all of the patients under the age of 30. The findings are reported in the December 2004 issue of the journal, Mayo Clinic Proceedings.

What diseases have been implicated due to Vitamin D Deficiency?

Alcoholism
Anxiety
Arthritis
Autoimmune diseases
Birth defects
Bone diseases
Bone pain
Burning in mouth
Cancer
Celiac-Sprue
Coeliac
Crohn's
Chronic Fatigue Syndrome
Chronic Pain
Cystic fibrosis
Depression
Diabetes
Diarrhea
Enzymatic diseases
Fatigue
Fibromyalgia
Graves' disease
Heart disease
Hernia
High blood pressure

Impaired wound healing
inflammatory bowel disease
Insomnia
Intestine
Irritability
Joint pain
Kidney
Liver
Lupus
Malabsorption
Multiple sclerosis
Muscle pain
Myopia
Nervousness
Obsessive Disorders
Osteomalacea
Osteoporosis
Panic Attacks
Parkinson's
Psoriasis
Rheumatoid arthritis
Rickets
Scalp sweating
Schizophrenia
Thyroid

Bob Barefoot On Vitamin-D

"The Cancer Inhibitor"

By

Robert R. Barefoot

© Copyright 2005
Robert R. Barefoot
Web Site "www.cureamerica.net"

Ode to Black America

By Bob Barefoot and Tim Matson

It's the time of our Lord, two thousand and five,

A time to wake up and all come alive.

Black America - still suffers - the most from disease,

While our medical leaders - praise their drug therapies.

Black Americans - now die - six years before Whites,

Giving up precious time – with no hope in sight.

As Black America succumbs - to cancer & disease

Their cry - has become - someone help us, PLEASE.

And their medical leaders do nothing about it ,

Except to stay quiet, so everyone will doubt it

For if Whites were dying - 6 years before Blacks do

Their leaders would spend billions, and you know that is true

There's no doubt they'd take action - to find what was wrong,

Lest people attack them - and think they weren't strong.

So this is our cause – and this is our plea

We must continue to fight - until we are <u>MEDICALLY FREE</u>.

Robert R. Barefoot

P.O. Box 21270
Wickenburg, Arizona 85358, U.S.A.
Phone 928-684-4458, Fax 928-684-8736
Email: "kingofcalcium@hotmail.com"
Web Site: "www.cureamerica.net"

Bob Barefoot on Vitamin-D
"The Cancer Inhibitor"

This publication is intended to direct the attention of both physician and patient to the scientific research being carried out concerning the significance of vitamin-D in regards to obtaining and sustaining optimal health. Due to irrefutable Scientific Research in conjunction with his own personal experience, it is Barefoot's opinion that vitamin-D supplementation can help to inhibit a whole host of diseases. This book is for educational purposes. It is not intended to replace the orthodox physician-patient relationship. If you are sick, you are advised to consult a physician, and together, along with your newly gained knowledge from this book, work towards the resolution of your illness.

Preliminary

This book is novel, new, controversial and thought provoking. Based on thirty years of personal research, Robert R. Barefoot, a renowned chemist, presents a powerful argument for the wide-ranging health benefits of vitamin-D supplementation. Steeped in mystery, folklore, credible testimonials and emerging science, this book describes how the common vitamin, vitamin-D is immerging as an almost potential cure-all to some of our most horrific diseases. However, if you are sick, you are advised to consult a physician, and together, along with your newly gained knowledge, work towards the resolution of your illness.

Referred to as "potentially toxic", there has never been a scientific study to prove this theory, while there have been several that prove just the opposite. Barefoot, who has been the champion of calcium health supplements (read his books **"The Calcium Factor"** and **"Let's Cure Humanity")** brings vitamin-D to the attention of Western society for its potential health benefits as a food supplement. Barefoot points to the massive amount of literature by the medical research community citing the health benefits of vitamin-D. He also points to the fact that to date the FDA has totally failed in its obligation to evaluate the potential of vitamin-D supplementation In spite of this fact, God gave us vitamin-D in several foods and biologically designed our bodies so that every time we expose our skin to UVB sunlight, we produce substantial quantities of this valuable nutrient. This God given biological function allows the human body to produce substantial quantities of this valuable nutrient every time we expose our skin to the sun.

Since 1982, Barefoot has watched as nutritional therapies have been used to help people cure themselves of disease when doctors said that there was no hope. The truth was that there was no hope as long as conventional medicine was applied, as *pharmaceutical drugs have never cured any degenerative disease.* However, God made the miraculous human body so that if it gets what it needs, it can heal itself. What the body needs is God's natural nutrition not white chemical killer drugs. The scientific community, on the other hand, has produced thousands of documents extolling vitamin-D's ability to alter disease. Therefore, the only hope to reverse the deadly course modern medicine has put on mankind is to begin the use of God's nutritional therapy.

Barefoot on Vitamin-D
"The Cancer Inhibitor"
By
Robert R. Barefoot
Published By:
Osa International Nutrition Ltd. Publishing
Post Office Box 21389
Wickenburg, AZ 85358 U.S.A.

All rights reserved. No part of this book may be reproduced or transmitted in any form or by any means, electronic or mechanical, including photocopying, recording or by any information storage and retrieval system without written permission from the author, except for the inclusion of brief quotations.

Copyright © 2005 by Robert R. Barefoot,
First Printing April, 2005

Library of Congress Cataloging in Publication Data
Barefoot, Robert R.
Barefoot on Vitamin-D,   The Cancer Inhibitor   by Robert R. Barefoot --- 1st edition
Bibliography
Includes subjects:
1. Biological Partners: Calcium& Vitamin-D
2. Scientific Quotations
3. Okinawa and Coral Calcium
4. Vitamin-D Toxicity
5. Vitamin-D and Black America

This book was not written to endorse the use of specific products or for any treatment purpose. The conclusions in this book represent the author's opinion of medical, scientific, folkloric and lay writings on the various topics discussed.

ISBN 0-9714224-1-9
Printed by RGM Management Services LLC.

Table of Contents

CONSUMER BEWARE !!!

Unbeknown to most Americans, we are being endangered by the ***pending avalanche of legislation*** which is being sponsored by the giant multinational drug companies. In April 1996, Congress passed, and the President signed into law, the **"Health Insurance Bill"**, which contains a rider from the ***World Health Organization Codex*** program that seeks to ***harmonize*** the governing and manufacture of health and medical products according to the standards set by the United Nations. The rider quietly passed. 90% of the Codex delegates represent ***multinational pharmaceutical corporations,*** mostly German, who are concerned about the potential encroachment of vitamins and minerals into their drug marketplace. Codex has proposed, and will soon have a mandate for the following guidelines for dietary supplements:

1. No dietary supplement can be sold for preventive use or therapeutic use.

2. No dietary supplement sold as food can exceed the potency levels set by the commission.

3. Codex regulations for dietary supplements would become binding.

4. All new dietary supplements would automatically be banned unless they go through the Codex approval process.

What this means is that, very soon, the Food and Drug Administration will have the authority to close down all health food stores and will require a medical doctor's prescription for vitamins, herbs and other supplements. The health of America will soon be turned over to the German drug industry, and America will not even have a vote. **At all cost, we must stop this from happening !!!**

Endorsements

"Mr. Barefoot is one of the Nation's top Nutritional Therapists, a chemist, scientist in the fields of biochemistry, hydrocarbon extraction and metal extraction from ores, inventor and holder of numerous patents, public speaker, writer, and outstanding business entrepreneur, a man of great integrity, enthusiasm, determination, loyalty, and tireless energy, coupled with a great personality. Mr. Barefoot has achieved wide acclaim in recent years for his biochemical research into the inter-relationship between disease and malnutrition, espousing that degenerative diseases are caused by mineral and vitamin deficiencies," Howard W. Pollock, Congressman (Alaska) Retired, Past President Safari Club International, Ducks Unlimited, and The National Rifle Association.

"I have been a practicing physician for the past 25 years. I am a fellow of the American College of OB-GYN and a diplomat of the American Board of OB-GYN. Mr. Barefoot has helped me immensely in understanding the complex chemistry of how calcium and other minerals contribute to overall health and preventive medicine. I personally know of many individuals who are much healthier today because of Mr. Barefoot's nutritional advice, including myself.," Wayne Weber M.D., Family Planning Associates Medical Group Inc., Los Angeles, California.

"I am a heart surgeon at Westchester Medical Center in Valhalla, New York, one of the largest open-heart surgery centers in the United States. I have had a special interest in nutrition over the past 30 years and have lectured on this subject throughout the United States, particularly its relationship to heart disease and other degenerative diseases. It is in this capacity that I have come to know and respect Robert Barefoot. He is an internationally known chemist with numerous international patents. His use of bio-chemistry in the field of hydrocarbon extraction and the field of metal extraction of ores led him to pursue a different line of research over the past two decades, elucidating the intimate relationship between nutrition and disease," Richard W. Pooley, Professor of Surgery, New York Medical College, New York.

*"I am a physician, President and Executive Medical Director of Health Insight, S.B.S. and Health Advocate Inc., in the State of Michigan. I have extensive credentials and honors that reach the White House and Heads of States in other countries. Mr. Robert Barefoot is a remarkable gentleman and a scholar who works endlessly to complete his mission to cure America. He has worked over the past 20 years with many medical doctors and scientists across the United States and in other countries doing Ortho- molecular Research on various diseases. The information has been culminated in two books, **'The Calcium Factor'** and **'Death by Diet'** which have been used technically as Bibles of Nutrition. Many people I know have thanked Mr. Barefoot for both saving their lives and returning them to good health. Mr. Barefoot is an amazing and extraordinary man who is on a 'Great Mission' for all mankind. I thank God for Robert Barefoot",* Liska M. Cooper, M.D., Detroit, Michigan

"I am a physician practicing at the Molecular/Biological level for over 25 years. I lecture extensively in the nutritional-medical field in Canada, the United states and internationally. I have attended hundreds of lectures and seminars covering the aspects of medicine including a number of those given by Robert Barefoot whose discourses easily classify as absolutely excellent. Personal conversations with this man, a highly moral and ethical person, have served to confirm his unusual knowledge in the field of biologically applied nutrition and immunity enhancement." C.T. Taylor, M.D., L.M.C.C., P. Eng., Stony Plain, Alberta.

"I have been an attorney involved in very complex litigation involving natural supplements and their ability to treat or cure various types of illnesses, including cancer. I am a well known in Maryland as a litigator, repeatedly being named as one of the outstanding trial attorneys, specializing in complex matters of all natures and have written concerning trial techniques. Mr. Barefoot was engaged as an expert in the use of natural supplements, specifically minerals, and their effect on various forms of cancers. He is a renowned author in this field. There have been many occasions when I found him to be extraordinarily knowledgeable in this field of expertise. My professional opinion is that Mr. Barefoot's knowledge and experience with minerals and other natural substances and their application for the treatment of illnesses is quite unique. In fact, I am not aware of any other individual who possesses the knowledge and expertise in this very important and expanding field as Mr. Barefoot," David Freishtat, Attorney, Freishtat & Sandler, Baltimore, Maryland.

*"Mr. Barefoot has been, and continues to be, an advocate for health and natural healing through nutrition and knowledge. He has championed the cause of well over 440,000 American women and children who have been exposed to the toxic effects of silicone implanted devices. Mr. Barefoot, one of the rare silica chemists in the world, has delivered a message of hope to these suffering individuals, who didn't have any hope before, but are now arming themselves with the books **The Calcium Factor** and **Death By Diet** and are spreading the word. The name Barefoot has become a household word. In the past three years, he has traveled to count-less meetings and medical conferences throughout the country without charging for his services. Robert Barefoot is a humanitarian and his efforts to educate through his books, informational tapes, lectures and vast media appearances has set a standard of excellence that is well above the norm. His work with hundreds of scientists and medical doctors, researching diet, has elevated him to one of the top speakers on nutrition in the nation,"* Jill M. Wood, President Idaho Breast Implant Information Group, Boise Idaho.

"I graduated from Harvard University in 1942 (BSC Chemistry) and worked as a Research Director and in corporate management, Franklin Electronics Inc., and have been awarded two patents. Mr. Barefoot has been highly influential in my survival of prostate cancer, with which I was diagnosed in the fall of 1991. Because of his detailed knowledge of biochemistry, he has much more penetrating knowledge of the relationship between disease and nutrition, a knowledge not available to many trained dieticians because of their lack of biochemical background. With his expertise, he has aided me in not only arresting the progression of my

disease, cancer, through diet and nutrition, but also reversing it. Mr. Barefoot is, simply put, an extraordinary individual," Philip Sharples, Sharples Industries Inc. Tubac, Arizona.

"I have known Bob Barefoot for three years during which time he has provided my spouse with critical information. As a result of this relationship, I was able to introduce dozens of people to Mr. Barefoot's idea relative to critical illness and nutrition. The results achieved have been remarkable. It is my personal opinion that Mr. Barefoot is the absolute top of his field, nutritional therapy," W. Grant Fairley, The Fairley Erker Group, Edmonton, Canada.

"I am a chemist and have been involved in product development, specifically nutritional supplements. I have written numerous articles and lectured throughout the United States on these products and the benefits of utilizing alternative medicine and alternative medical products within the U.S. healthcare regimen. Over the past three years I have traveled and lectured with Mr. Barefoot on numerous occasions all over the United States. He is recognized as a world class expert on calcium and its nutritional benefits for the human body. Mr. Barefoot blends his prestige and uncanny ability to talk to the average person in a way that allows complicated scientific subjects to be completely understandable and accepted. I have seen Mr. Barefoot's information help a lot of people," Alex Nobles, Executive Vice President, Benchmark USA Inc., Salt Lake.

"I have been associated with Mr. Barefoot since 1993. His Nutrition therapy is the result of twenty years of research

into non-invasive treatment of generic diseases. In Canada we now have six M.D.'s practicing his protocols. I understand that numerous Russian M.D.'s in Moscow are also practicing his protocols. This number will increase exponentially as the testimonial success of hundreds of afflicted people becomes known. Mr. Barefoot's biochemistry and science brings credence to his recommended dietary and lifestyle protocols. He must be considered at the top of his field," Peter Epp. P. Eng., President Albritco Development Corporation, Calgary, Canada.

"I am the General Manager of an audio cassette tape manufacturer. Previously, I was the Vice President of an engineering consulting company specializing in nuclear technology analysis under contract to the U.S. government. With a BS degree in Electrical Engineering, graduate school work at UCLA and over 10 years of research at McDonnell Douglas; my technical and scientific tools are extensive. I currently specialize in the audio production of technical information specializing in nutrition and health. It is in this regard that I have come to know the reputation and work of Robert Barefoot. Our company actively seeks men and women with scientific and medical backgrounds in order to develop substantive resource material for our client base. Robert Barefoot's lectures, books and tapes support his position as a leading spokesperson for the benefits of nutrition for good health," Al Vendetti, General Manager, Exxel Audio Productions, Ocean-side, California.

"I am the founder of a company that specializes in both mining and the export of health and nutritional products overseas. Mr. Barefoot has tremendous knowledge of

biochemistry and his expertise in the field of calcium research has earned him recognition worldwide for both his lecturing and his research. He has authored several books which my company exports overseas as nutritional standards for people involved in the nutrition industry. He has also researched and developed calcium supplements, which are being exported to several countries abroad. His research of the relationship between disease and nutrition is gaining recognition worldwide and, if properly implemented, could substantially reduce the devastating effects of degenerative diseases caused by mineral and vitamin deficiency," Brett R. Davies, President, Davies International, Denver, Colorado.

"I am well known in the area of nutrition. I am certified by the National Association of Health Care Professionals as a Health Care Councilor and have lectured extensively in the United States, Canada, Russia and the Ukraine. Mr. Barefoot is considered one of the most knowledgeable people in the world, on effects of calcium on health", Robert G. Bremner, Mechanicsville, Virginia.

"Mr. Barefoot is a man in pursuit of "Excellence" in all his endeavors. He has received wide recognition for his research in the biochemistry field, dealing with malnutrition. I have the distinct privilege and pleasure of having known Mr. Barefoot for several years". **Jerry R. Gallion, International Financier, Vaulx Milieu, France.**

"I am a retired university professor, Ph.D., known in the field of Pharmaceutical Chemistry, having written and lectured extensively over a forty year period, publishing numerous scientific articles. Based on Mr. Barefoot's education, and background in chemistry and nutrition, along with his published books and lecturing, it is my professional opinion that Mr. Barefoot is near the top of his field".
Jerry Rollins, PhD., Austin, Texas.

We have purchased two of your books, "The Calcium Factor" and "Death ByDiet". INCREDIBLE BOOK!!! Well worth reading by EVERY PERSON IN AMERICA OF READING AGE!! I HAVE READ THEM TWICE.

We totally discount the crap that the "fanatics" in other fields and in the government who discount your writings. <u>*It does show how afraid they are of the TRUTH, doesn't it?*</u> *Bob we feel that your sales of coral calcium have helped so many people (including ourselves) and should continue unabated. Our congratulations to you for writing the EXCELLENT information you have in those books, and, therefore, helping to benefit many, many, many people's health.*

We wish unabated success for you continuing your writings, work and success in defeating the scared idiots.
Mae and Al Schone, Felton PA.

*"As a result of reading **The Calcium Factor** I received excellent treatment and eventually cured myself of prostate cancer. I strongly endorse Mr. Barefoot as one of the top people in his area having excellent knowledge of nutritional therapy. I have yet to find anyone who has written such well-reasoned and scientifically based material,"* David G McLean, Chairman of the Board, Canadian National Railways."

*"In October 1996 I was diagnosed with prostate cancer. The diagnosis was confirmed by biopsy. In October of that year I started following Robert Barefoot's calcium regime. In July 1997 I had another prostate biopsy in which no evidence of malignancy was found. The regime outlined in the book **The Calcium Factor** improves the immune system to where the body can heal itself, without intrusive measures like surgery, chemotherapy or radiation,"* S. Ross Johnson, Retired President of Prudential Insurance Company of America.

Preface

For over two decades, Bob Barefoot has been known as a *medical maverick*, because of his choice to both live and research preventive medicine. He is not a stranger to controversy and debate. Having started his career in pure chemistry and related sciences, he became fascinated by the bigger picture on how physical science can explain many aspects of the complexities of biological systems. The turning point in his career was his interaction with the late Dr. Carl Reich MD, first as a scientist and subsequently as a collaborative researcher. The wisdom of Dr. Carl Reich's observations (upon his death a few years ago, Dr. Reich was referred to as *"The Father of Preventive Medicine"*) on the importance of calcium and vitamin-D for health attracted much debate. In fact his revolutionary proposals on the role of calcium with vitamin-D as a versatile and potent biological combination that can prevent and treat many diseases were so challenging to his peers that he suffered oppression, rejection and ridicule while his patients were experiencing almost miraculous cures. Then, in 1984 Dr. Carl Reich lost his license *"for claiming that calcium supplements cure cancer"*, a claim that is now echoed by many of our best medical researchers today. Just prior to his death, City Scope magazine in Calgary did a feature article entitled *"Ahead of His Time"*, in which they credit Dr. Reich with the passage of

Bill #209, the Province of Alberta Medical Profession Amendment Act, which states that *"a practitioner shall not be found guilty of unbecoming conduct or found to be incapable or unfit to practice medicine solely on the basis that the practitioner employs a therapy that is non-traditional or departs from the prevailing medical practices, unless it can be demonstrated by medical authorities that the therapy has a safety risk for that patient unreasonably greater than the prevailing treatment"*.

$\quad$The History of medicine is replete with examples of the hazards that scientists face when they propose a theory that may not be palatable to prevailing bodies of opinion. Dr. Reich showed, by a lifetime of practical treatment experience, that vitamin-D with calcium and other minerals play a vital role in the biology of life. In the 1960's he collaborated with Dr. Otto Warburg, two time Nobel Prize winner, to write a book on the subject, but Warburg died prior to completion. Dr. Warburg lectured to American students in 1966 stating that *"there was no disease that we know more about the cause or the cure than cancer, but because of the agnostics in the AMA and FDA, millions of Americans would have to die needlessly"*.

$\quad$Since he gave this warning, over 25,000,000 Americans have died needlessly. They were your loved ones, your relatives, your friends. While we would like to believe that modern science is more open to *"new"* suggestions or *"reactivated interest"* in rejected theories, the modern-day questioning of the prevailing bodies of medical opinion seems to be equally as hazardous for many researchers as it was several centuries ago. Albert Einstein said it best, *"great spirits have always encountered violent opposition from mediocre minds".*

The phenomenon of the *"lone hero against the world"* is sometimes used as an excuse to gain unjustified support for alternative scientific thoughts, but powerful economic influences act against the obvious introduction of simple natural options for health maintenance. Healthcare in the West is dominated by allopathic (conventional) thinking which tends to focus on pharmaceutical developments and classical surgical strategies. The incentives to engage in preventive medicine are not as powerful as those to treat established disease with proprietary technology that generates staggering profits. Fortunately modern medicine is changing as more individuals demand alternatives. Some conventional approaches to disease prevention or treatment may on occasion result in dubious success.

The title of this book **"Barefoot on Vitamin-D"** tells a story. Barefoot stands for vitamin-D as being a unique and valuable bio nutrient for health as well as, in his opinion, the best vitamin supplement available. Vitamin-D is a *"powerhouse of health"* giving nutrient supplementation that combines to support all body chemistry.

This book on vitamin-D is the culmination of three decades of research. There are several communities through-out the world that enjoy health and longevity to a greater degree than humankind. The common denominator in this phenomenon is not their sedentary lifestyle and the fact that they eat fish, fruits and vegetables. **Many cultures live nearby and do the same but do not have the same health**

18

benefits, but rather it is the abundant mineral supply in their diet, especially calcium. The fact is that they all receive several hours daily of direct sunshine that produces an abundance of vitamin-D for the body to defend itself. As a result, the vitamin-D allows for the increased absorption of Calcium due to vitamin-D lining the VDR receptors of the intestinal wall. The inhabitants of Okinawa in Japan are one example of this status of *"super health and well-being"*. Ask yourself a simple question, would you be surprised if an outdoor plant or shrub with daily exposure to the sun, grew better, lived longer & looked healthier than a plant that is indoors without any exposure to direct sunlight? Of course not! So, why would the human body be any different?

In an article in the January 1973 edition of **National Geographic** entitled *"Search For The Oldest People"* provided examples of many of these cultures including the **Abkhasians** from Georgia (high in the mountains), the **Hunzas** of Pakistan (high in the mountains), and the **Vilcabambas** of Ecuador (high in the mountains). This list can be quickly expanded to include the **Bamas** in China (high in the mountains), the **Azerbaijans** (high in the mountains), the **Armenians** (high in the mountains), the **Tibetans** (high in the mountains), and the **Titicacas** of Peru (high in the mountains). To this list, of course the Okinawans of Japan (sea level) must be added. *It is interesting to note that all of these cultures are outdoor cultures who receive several hours daily of direct sunshine resulting in the production of substantial vitamin-D.*

As noted above, other than the Okinawans, each of these long living cultures live at high elevations. *Recent clinical research has proven UVB exposure at higher altitudes stimulates not only a greater production of vitamin D but also increases the rate of sunburn* compared to sea level UVB exposure. One study suggested, for example, *that an average complexion burns at six minutes at 11,000 feet at noon compared to 25 minutes at sea level in a temperate climate.* This means that at high solar elevations the ratio favors vitamin-D formation. At lower solar altitudes, it may be impossible to form vitamin-D without sunburning depending on the amount of skin surface exposed. (Effects of Solar Altitude -vs- Artificial Spectra on Vitamin D & Erythema)

With all of the above cultures, *disease virtually does not exist: "almost"* no cancer, no heart disease, no diabetes, no Alzheimer's, no arthritis, etc. For example, the Okinawans have less that one fifth the heart disease that Americans do. These cultures have no mental disorders and no doctors. They also live much longer than we do in North America and their aging process is dramatically slower. For example the Okinawans live 8 years longer than mainland Japan residents who lives 4 years longer than Americans. And the elderly seem to have youthful bodies. *The common denominator is that all are sun loving cultures and that all of their water is loaded with mineral nutrients from melting glaciers high in the mountains, and from the disintegrating coral reefs in Okanawa.* One quart of Hunza water, in Pakistan, contains 17,000 milligrams of calcium (42 times the RDA), which is also equivalent to 17 quarts of milk, and they drink several quarts each day. In general, the over-riding factor in their disease-free longevity is the fact that these cultures can consume almost *"one hundred times the RDA"* of everything (except for the sun, however they get many times more sunshine than the typical American) with the only side effect being great health and longevity. Also, they consume large amounts of everything that we are told is not good for us such as sunshine, butter, salt, eggs, milk and animal fat.

The major beneficial factor which can not be disputed is the fact that these cancer-free people are *sun loving*, which we are told causes cancer. While many Africans spend most of every day *naked in the sun* and are almost completely *cancer-free*, Black Americans, with the same genes, who avoid the sun like the plague, are ravished by cancer and are almost at double the risk of cancer as are White Americans who sun bathe. Barefoot and Dr. Reich wrote the book, **"The Calcium Factor"** which detailed the scientific explanations for this cancer phenomenon and for the remarkable health and youth of others. The book was published in 1992. Mr. Barefoot was immediately invited as a guest speaker at health shows and was a frequent guest on numerous radio and television talk shows. Ten years later, in 2002, he was to make of the most watched infomercials in television history, having a dramatic impact on nutrition in America.

It is hoped that when you read this book you will discover the reasoning behind vitamin-D and minerals for good health. Bob Barefoot believes that this truth will one day help cure humanity.

Acknowledgement

The author is grateful and wishes to acknowledge his appreciation for the dedication, contributions and efforts of Fay Harlin, Barney Woods, John Baker his friend and wife Isabelle, Bruce and Carole Downey, Tim Matson for his insight, his love of the truth, tenacious assistance and for inspiring the writing of this book, and most of all, his cherished wife of 36 years, Karen Barefoot, in assisting the completion, critical review and editing of this publication.

Notation

Although this publication is intended to direct the attention of both the physician and the patient to the torrent of scientific research being carried out on the significance of vitamin-D, it is not the intention of the authors to provide an alternative to the orthodox physician-patient relationship. Rather, it is the objective of the authors to expand the dimensions of orthodox medicine itself, and help speed it towards medical practices of the twenty-first century where diet and lifestyle will play a predominant role in preventive medicine.

"If the doctors of today do not become the nutritionists of tomorrow, the nutritionists of today will become the doctors of tomorrow." (Rockefeller Institute of Medical Research).

CHAPTER ONE

Black America First

Because so many people who are in suffering and pain have sought my help, I have become passionate about ending degenerative disease. I have seen the success of using God's nutrients and I know that the results can be explained in detail in scientific terms. ***Both God and Science are one in the same.*** However, if we start to cure disease we should start with those most affected, the Black American community in the United States. Black America suffers from highest cancer rates of all ethnic groups, almost twice as much s whites **(American Cancer Society: *"Cancer Facts and Figures for African Americans 2004-2005", Blacks have approximately 30 to 40% more cancer and in some cases a 250% higher death rate than Whites*)** twice the diabetes and five times the kidney disease, and diseases whites have not heard of, such as sickle cell anemia. And even more tragically, **life expectancy for Black men is 68.6 years old** compared to 75.0 for White men(6.4 year difference) and **Black women are 75.5** versus 80.2 for White women (4.7Year Difference) (**American Cancer Society,**

"Cancer Facts and Figures for African Americans 2004-2005). This is a *"six year discrepancy"* for men and almost a *five year discrepancy* for women that just makes me want to scream!!!

In my life, I have never seen a worse form of racial prejudice. Millions of Blacks have died prematurely, in pain and needlessly. If white Americans were dying six years before the Blacks and suffered from twice as much disease, the regulatory authorities would be spending hundreds of billions of dollars to find out why. These same agencies, the FDA, the FTC and the AMA have not spent one dime on the Blacks. Why??? The only answer can be racial prejudice. Because of my passion on this subject, many in the Black American community have tried to get Oprah Winfrey to talk to me, but unfortunately, she has a wall of protection around her that decides for her what she should hear. If she would one day be able to listen, my message to her would be, *"Let's cure humanity, starting with Black America a first."*

In Chapter Twelve, **"Vitamin-D and Black America",** the direct relationship of the epidemic vitamin-D deficiency among Black Americans and this health discrepancy will be explained. This is very troubling because the elderly are also at extreme risk for vitamin-D deficiency and it has been observed that 30% of free-living elderly whites, 42% of elderly Hispanics, and *84% of elderly Blacks* were vitamin-D deficient in a study performed in Boston. (*"Vitamin-D: Importance in the Prevention of Cancers, Type 1 Diabetes, Heart Disease, and Osteoporosis"*) *From the Vitamin-D Skin and Bone Research Laboratory, Section of Endocrinology, Diabetes and Nutrition, Department of*

Medicine, Boston University School of Medicine, Boston MA).

I would like to challenge each and every celebrity in America to look, listen and learn, and then to do what is right as America will eagerly follow you. You therefore have the ability to end suffering and misery in America. All you have to do is to try God's nutrients after you read this book. Almost every American who tries the nutrient program notices a difference. Those who are sick, of course, notice the most. Many who were given only weeks to live are now healthy. Some, who were in wheel chairs, are now able to walk. Many Americans are starting to discover the magic of using God's nutrients instead of white chemical drugs. However, most Americans still believe that there is no hope, and this list includes almost all celebrities who are protected by the well meaning establishment. Unfortunately, this means that they are protected until their premature deaths.

Steve McQueen did not have to die according to Dr Otto Warburg. I know this to be true. The same is true for Michael Landon, John Wayne, and Jerry Orbach. The list goes on and on, and every American can add others to this list. All Americans loved these guys and now they are all dead. They died needlessly. They died in pain. I cried for them all, and yet all could have been saved. My children begged me to contact them but I could not get behind their barriers.

I did try but they were so protected by security that their only chance for survival was prevented from happening. We have to break down the barrier to let these desperate people know that neither their pain nor their death is eminent. They can live!!! But this can never happen until the celebrities in America wake up and learn that there is indeed an alternative. Until this happens they will continue suffering and dying needlessly. I hope to one day soon have a Barefoot in Hollywood party for celebrities so I can educate them on how to live & thrive. They will learn about coral calcium and gladly agree to sunbathe. We can save them all !!!

Like most of America, watching celebrities die needlessly breaks my heart when I know they could be saved. We have to get celebrities to listen, to learn and to try. We need the assistance from the powerful public leaders of Black America like Oprah Winfrey and Jesse Jackson to help us get this information to the people who are suffering the most. I have had dozens of Americans tell me that they will get to Oprah. All have failed!!! All Americans should solicit their favorite celebrity. If they succeed, in the end they will be saving lives. The cost is only a few cents a day, so money is not a factor.

I believe that after you read this book and try the program for yourself, you will be totally sold. If you love your country, you will join me in my efforts to **Cure America.** Then, when the celebrities try the program, they will discover the magic. If they are willing to tell their fellow Americans, the average American will gladly listen and follow their example because they are celebrities. The result will be that the celebrities will have helped to create a disease-free America. They owe it to their country to try.

CHAPTER TWO

<u>VITAMIN-D AND KIDS</u>

As a kid I learned in elementary school that the dreaded disease rickets was cured when they discovered that it was caused by a vitamin-D deficiency. We were told that as a result, all milk was fortified with vitamin-D, wiping out this horrific disease known as rickets.

Of course we were told that you could also get vitamin-D from certain foods such as eggs and fish. We were also told that the body produces its own vitamin-D every time it is exposed to sunshine. Thus, even as kids we had to conclude that rickets was caused by lack of sunshine on the skin. Today, a whole host of other diseases, including cancer, Diabetes & Heart Disease has been added to the list.

A newborn's vitamin-D is approximately one-half that of its mother's vitamin-D. A risk factor for poor vitamin-D status in early infancy is maternal vitamin-D deficiency during pregnancy, resulting in inadequate maternal transfer of vitamin-D to the fetus and low infant stores. *Infants and young children who are vitamin-D deficient may be imprinted for the rest of their lives with increased risk of type 1 diabetes multiple sclerosis, rheumatoid arthritis, and many common cancers.* Recently it has been reported that young adults with vitamin-D deficiency were at greater risk of congestive heart failure than were their vitamin-D sufficient counterparts. (*"Vitamin-D: Importance in the Prevention of Cancers, Type 1 Diabetes, Heart Disease, and Osteoporosis",* Department of Medicine, Boston University School of Medicine).

The fact that there is a long list of diseases caused by vitamin-D deficiency is particularly disturbing as today we are also told by the medical *"experts"* that the sun is the cause of some cancers, because as we all know, some people (not all) who aggravate their skin with sunburns, do indeed develop skin cancers during their lifetime. Therefore we slather our kids with sun block to protect them from cancer. In effect, what the doctors are saying is that God must have made a mistake when he gave us the sun. In reality, it is the doctors who are making the mistakes as there are many scientific studies that now prove that the sun actually protects us against most cancers, as you will see in Chapter 6, *Scientific Quotations.* In the meantime, these *"experts"* continue to try to develop a white chemical drug that will prevent disease and make the men of medicine rich.

It is foolish to propose that any single agent will promote health and longevity in a consistent and simple manner. After all, aging and disease development are highly complex biological events with a multitude of contributory factors. However, it should be noted that vitamin-D cannot be considered a *"single agent"*, but rather a necessary and crucial ingredient of human health. Man did not make this compound. God did!!! The problem is that the drug industry with its puppet government agencies such as the FDA, AMA and FTC all mislead the American public to believe that they are very close to producing the wonder drug to eliminate disease and prolong life. The truth is that in the past 100 years of trying, all of these agencies have failed miserably. They have not cured or prevented *"one"* degenerative disease from occurring. *Not one!!!* They have eliminated polio, but polio is not a degenerative disease like cancer or diabetes, it is caused by a virus, and they know how to handle viruses. But when it comes to the diseases that are killing us, like cancer at 3% in 1900, 20% in 1950 and almost 40% in 2000, the drug industry with its puppet government agencies have failed miserably. If the trend continues we will all suffer a painful premature death.

The problem is that the medical authorities are doing nothing different, and they have a vested interest in maintaining the status quo (and their profits), so anything that jeopardizes this position is attacked with all of the might of the government. This means that when the medical researchers suggest that vitamin-D could inhibit cancer, the press does not report it, not to mention the fact that doctors are told by the drug industry that vitamin-D is toxic.

Medical researchers tell us that vitamin-D inhibits and reverses a host of diseases (see quotes to follow) implying that cancer, for example can be *"cured"*. *Can you imagine what would happen if they said the same about any particular drug.* That drug would instantly be worth trillions of dollars. Ironically, medical researchers are indeed saying the same thing about many of God's other nutrients, such as calcium (see quotes to follow). *They are virtually saying that God's nutrients, vitamin-D and calcium can indeed both cure and prevent cancer and a host of other degenerative diseases.* Many medical quotes will be given later in Chapter 6, However, one example will now be given below.

Ken C. Chiu, Oct 16, 2004, Vol 166, #16, Page248 University of California, Los Angeles School of Medicine May 1 American Journal of Clinical Nutrition.

"Vitamin D may play a role in the prevention of diabetes as well as of cancer. Many studies have linked vitamin D deficiency to an increased risk of type 2 diabetes, which used to be called adult-onset diabetes".

"Vitamin D deficiency is a <u>double jeopardy for type 2 diabetes."</u> concludes Chiu. He says he now "worries that for people on the cusp of developing the disease, vitamin deficiency may tip the balance."

http://www.diabetes.org/diabetes-statistics.jsp

Setting these technical thoughts aside, humankind has not only been searching for a potion to cure diseases associated with aging, but it has also been on a perpetual search for one potion, lotion or elixir that will guarantee eternal youth. While this miracle eludes discovery by the drug industry, some of the secrets of health and longevity may be much more simple than hitherto supposed, as simple as the one-two combination of the biological partners calcium and vitamin-D.

CHAPTER THREE

<u>VITAMIN-D</u>

<u>AND ETERNAL YOUTH</u>

Implicit in the desire for eternal youth is our wish to avoid poor health which seems to emerge with advancing age. Of all the interventions that have been tried for enhancing well-being and long-life, few have worked. I believe that the issues are tied up in our lifestyle. The biblical patriarchs, who definitely had a different lifestyle, lived to be over 900 years old. Today, a healthy lifestyle is a key factor in extending life that must have the quality of being free from disease. Beyond the important obvious issues like health sermons on cigarette smoking, stress, drug abuse etc., nutritional factors figure most strongly as determinants of health and well-being. The avoidance of all destructive behavior is advisable, but the domain of lifestyle most amenable to correction is *"sound and appropriate nutrition including sunshine"*.

It is easy for a chemist (like myself) to see the body as a <u>universe</u> of interacting chemicals. While this perception provides an incomplete picture of life, it is a good start to understanding the importance of vitamins and minerals as a vital component of a diet for health, as each mineral must serve at least one specific biological function. With the exception of aluminum and silicon, the human body is made up of the same minerals, <u>including gold,</u> in differing amounts as the Earth. I shall present evidence that mineral balance (especially calcium) in the body along with vitamins is an absolute prerequisite for health and longevity, but I trust this important advice will be taken in conjunction with a healthy lifestyle.

"**L**ongevity" is ultimately determined by the time of death. Within this term is the implication of quality of life. This means that longevity is viewed as the length of time that one can live under the most favorable circumstances. The quest for longevity involves the retention of health. In Western society, ill health is often considered to be inevitable with advancing years. Our aim is to move away from this circumstance and toward longer life expectancy associated with quality of life. In Okinawa health and a long life seem to go together, which is the same for all of the other cultures around the world that experience good health and longevity. Why? This is a question that begs to be answered!!!

One might be impressed by media reports that we are living longer. In actuality, recently human life span has not increased dramatically and in fact lags far behind the experiences of Okinawans and other cultures that exhibit longevity (e.g. Vilacambans, Abkhasians and Hunzukats). I stress that the *"factor common to all"* of these people seems to be the **generous supply of minerals and elements in their environment and their daily exposure to generous amounts of sunlight which stimulates vitamin-D production.** Each culture consumes what a Western doctor would consider a staggering and lethal amount of minerals (such as calcium: up to 100,000 milligrams daily). Yet, these people do not die prematurely, as they lead exceedingly long and healthy lives while the Western doctor's patients, following his advice, die young and usually in pain.

The secret of why these people do not age is that their telomeres do not break down. A telomere is a repeated DNA sequence found at the end of chromosomes that protect the chromosome from disintegration. At birth telomeres consist of about 15,000 base pairs of repeated sequences, which become shorter with cell division. Every time a cell divides it loses 25 to 200 DNA base pairs off the telomer ends. Once this pruning has occurred about 100 times the cell ages and does not continue dividing, so we grow old fast.

Dr. S Benet published his observation on longevity factors in a book entitled **"How to live to be 100"** (The Dial Press, NY 1976). In the book Dr. Benet reported major differences in the dietary patterns of long living people compared with those with a shorter life span. Similar observations were made by Dr. D. Davis who studied the lifestyle habits and environment of centenarians who live at high altitudes in the Andes Mountains of South America (Davis D, **The Centenarians of the Andes**, Double Day Publishing Co, NY, 1975). Also, Dr. Allen E Bank, who studied the famous *Hunzas* of Northern Pakistan discovered and reported in his book **Hunza Land,** that their diet was substantially different, and that they ate their food immediately upon harvest or slaughter, and never peeled or skinned their fruits or vegetables. He also noted that they always ate the animal organs, including the delicacy of intestine full of vegetation. He further noted that they ate several foods that were "very high in *calcium* content", such as soybean flour (330mg/cup), molasses (116mg/tsp), goat's milk (305mg/8oz), kale (450mg/cup), bone meal (610mg/cup), and almonds (572mg/cup). And remember that there water contains 17,000 milligrams of calcium per quart.

Dr, Benet also quoted Douglas Spies, M.D., a recipient of the **A.M.A. Distinguished Services Award**, who in 1959 in a talk to the members of the American Medical Association said *"All disease is caused by chemicals, and all disease can be cured by chemicals"* (Note: Dr. Hippocrates, Father of Medicine declared *'All food is medicine and the best food is the best medicine'*). *All the chemicals used by the body are taken in through food. If we only knew enough, all disease could be prevented and could be cured through proper nutrition."* Why won't doctors listen???

We therefore can listen to the experts or we can learn from the experiences of the inhabitants of Okinawa who are one of the healthiest and longest living people in the world. They have ten times as many centenarians per area found in the United States and large numbers of robust individuals in their eighties and nineties. When in their 80's, their body parts are as youthful as men and women in their twenties & thirties.

While many factors may operate to create this desirable circumstance, I, like the Spanish explorers before me and the Japanese scientists of today, believe a key to this circumstance is the use of coral calcium as a food supplement in this highly blessed community of people. In addition, it should be noted that the human intestine is lined with vitamin-D receptors known as VDR's. *When the VDR's are full of vitamin-D (about 5000IU vitamin-D is required for this) then the intestine is capable of absorbing 2000% more calcium.* Therefore, if the coral calcium is going to keep the Okinawans youthful, then vitamin-D is required. *This necessitates the exposure of their skin to the sun,* which, because they are an outdoor society, is no problem for the Okinawans.

While some people may dismiss this phenomenon as a chance observation, there are new scientific and medical discoveries that give a credible, scientific basis for the use of coral calcium for health. One key constituent of coral calcium is readily absorbable calcium and magnesium, but other factors within coral, including its highly balanced mineral content and the occurrence of microbes, may account for observed benefits. Oprah Winfrey recently had "experts" on her show that said that the reason for the longevity and good health of the Okinawans was the good food they eat and their lifestyles. Although this sounds acceptable, it does not stand the test of scientific scrutiny or even simple logic. Only a short distance away from Okinawa there are islands where the people eat the same food, have the same lifestyle and yet they are diseased and have a much shorter life expectancy. Also, prestigious Japanese scientists have concluded that the reason for the good health and longevity of the Okinawan people is their consumption of *'calcium rich coral water'*.

However, despite recent findings, for a great many years, Japanese and American scientists and researchers attributed longevity in Okinawa Prefecture to the climate and diet of the people. This is an obvious misconception that can be proven. In Okinawa, the one thing that we are certain of is that for many years Okinawans have used coral in inventive ways and even when not added in their food preparation, its habitual presence enriches the environment largely through its presence in water. Then in the 1950's Professor Jun Kobayashi revealed his "ground-breaking" work that showed *"a direct relationship between the 'hard water' that is consumed by Okinawans and their long and healthy life span."* The work of Professor Kobyashi was published in The Sokai journal of Okinawa under the loosely translated title *"The secret of health and longevity in Okinawa, where many people live to an advanced age and where the incidence of all diseases is low"*. Also, in 1985, Dr. Jun Sato, Professor of Okayama University presented his research at the academic society where his investigation concluded that the lower rate of disease and the longevity of the Okinawans *"was due to the calcium enriched coral water"*. Finally, Professor Jun Kobayashi of the University of Okayama presented a paper in 1990 where *"he concluded that there was a correlation between longevity and good health and the calcium rich coral water in Okinawa"*. Thus, the men of science in Japan have all concluded that the good health and longevity of the Okinawans is due to the calcium rich coral waters, which means that vitamin-D, working in biological tandem with calcium due to its assistance in its absorption in the intestine, also plays a crucial role in the fountain of youth.

CHAPTER FOUR

<u>Vitamin D Food Sources</u>

Table 1, Best Food Sources for Vitamin-D

fatty fish such as salmon, cooked, 3.5 oz.....360 IU

mackerel, cooked, 3.5 oz.......................345 IU

sardines, canned in oil, drained, 3.5 oz........270 IU

eel, cooked, 3.5 oz.............................200 IU

fish oils such as cod liver oil, 1 Tbs.........1,360 IU

egg yolk (one whole yolk)........................25 IU

Did you know Government Agencies (USDA) don't list naturally occurring vitamin-D Levels in these food sources. This is intentional because of the high levels of vitamin-D in Fish. We all know that Fish is very good for us so they can't list the vitamin-D levels that naturally occur in fish or they would have to raise their RDA levels for supplements.

If large amounts of vitamin-D are available from fish and fish oils, then fish must require large amounts of vitamin-D in their diets, as well as the associated minerals.

Vitamins

The vitamins are generally defined as dietary essential organic compounds, required only in minute amounts, and which play a catalytic role and but no major structural role. *So far, 4 fat-soluble and 11 water-soluble vitamins or vitamin-like compounds have been shown to be essential to fish.* Requirement is generally measured in young fast growing fish. However, requirements may depend on the intake of other nutrients, size of the fish, and environmental stress. The recommended levels and the deficiency signs are summarized in Tables 2 and 3. Nutritional disorders caused by vitamin deficiencies can impair utilization of other nutrients, impair the health of fish, and finally lead to disease or deformities.

Minerals

Inorganic elements (minerals) are required by fish for various functions in metabolism and osmoregulation. Fish obtain minerals from their diet but also from their environment. Many minerals are required in trace amounts and are present in sufficient quantity in the surrounding water for the fish to absorb through their gills. In freshwater, there is generally sufficient concentration of calcium, sodium, potassium and chloride for the fish to absorb and cover its requirements. The totality of the requirement for other minerals must, in general, be covered by the diet. The recommended levels of minerals in the diet are shown in Table 2. Reduced growth, feed efficiency and skeletal deformities is the most common signs of mineral deficiencies.

Table 2. Vitamin requirement of salmonids.

Vitamin	Requirement
Fat-soluble vitamins	
Vitamin A, IU/kg	2,500
Vitamin D, IU/kg	**2,400**
Vitamin E, IU/kg	50
Vitamin K, mg/kg	1
Water-soluble vitamin, mg/kg	
Riboflavin	4
Pantothenic acid	20
Niacin	10
Vitamin B12	0.01
Biotin	0.15
Folate	1.0
Thiamin	1
Vitamin B6	3
Vitamin C	50
Vitamin-like compounds, mg/kg	
Choline	1,000

Table 3. Mineral requirement of salmonid fish in fresh water.

Mineral	Requirement (mg/kg feed)*
Calcium (Ca)	10,000
Chlorine (Cl)	9,000
Potassium (K)	7,000
Sodium (Na)	6,000
Phosphorus (P)	6,000
Magnesium (Mg)	500
Iron (Fe)	60
Zinc (ZN)	30
Manganese (MN)	13
Copper (Cu)	3
Iodine (I)	1.1
Selenium (Se)	0.3

*Requirement in the absence of significant amounts of the specific mineral in the water.

Thus, in order to be healthy, it is evident that fish, just like people, require both large amounts of calcium and vitamin-D in their diet. The calcium for fish comes from the environmental waters and the vitamin-D must come from sunshine & photosynthesis. Fortunately for people, much of our required vitamin-D and calcium comes from eating the fish, after they have absorbed these nutrients.

CHAPTER FIVE

BIOLOGICAL PARTNERS

WHY CALCIUM? WHY VITAMIN-D?

Every time we turn on the radio we hear that calcium is good for you. All foods are being stuffed with calcium. Television is also full of the same advertising telling us that calcium is good for us, but no one will tell us why, other than it makes us healthy. But How??? And Why ???

Also, if indeed calcium is so good for us, *then its biological partner, vitamin-D, must be just as good, but no one is extolling the virtues of vitamin-D.* One thing for sure is that the American public needs to be told in simple terms why and how these nutrients make us healthy.

The answer, ironically, is indeed simple. First, there is more calcium in the human body than any other mineral. It is involved in hundreds of biological functions crucial to life. Excess calcium is stored in the bones to replenish calcium levels when the body is calcium deficient in order to perform its crucial biological functions. However, to maintain health, this bone calcium must be replaced, and unfortunately, calcium is one of the hardest minerals for the body to absorb. So, where should you get your calcium?

Of course in the beginning it is mother's milk, from which much of her immunity to disease is also transferred to the infant. Then, because we are not animals who will eat bushels of calcium rich grass, most of us get our calcium from cows' milk. But, as we get older we drink less and less milk, and many of us shy away from dairy products, meaning that our bones slowly become depleted in calcium.

But, that is not all that happens. When the body has adequate calcium, it has an ability to ward off disease and to maintain youth. Wow!!! That is a big claim, and fortunately, it has been proven by the scientific community, as will be seen in the chapter on scientific quotations.

The human intestine is lined with human *vitamin-D receptors* known as *VDR's*. These VDR's are also present in the bone and kidney as well as in the parathyroid glands. *When the VDR's are full of vitamin-D (about 5000IU vitamin-D is required for this)   then the intestine is capable of absorbing 2000% more calcium.* "VDR's are also found in the melanoma cells, breast carcinoma cells and osteo-sarcoma cells where vitamin-D *inhibits the proliferation of cancer as well as in the pancreas* where vitamin-D enhances the production of insulin; in the heart muscle where vitamin-D enhances ventricular contractility; and in many other organs where it plays a *crucial biological role."* The American Public must be made aware of the **1-2 punch** provided by **the biological partners Calcium & vitamin-D** and the scientific fact that **they must be taken in conjunction with one another.**

In 1972, Albert Lehniger, Professor of Medical Science, John Hopkins University) made a major scientific discovery. *He discovered that DNA, the body's blueprint for repair to correct damage and keep us young, would only work when smothered in calcium.* Thus, calcium became indispensable for body repair. In his book, "**The Role of Calcium Biological Systems,** which is a compilation of dozens of scientific publications by academically recognized scientists, he writes that there is a link between calcium deficiency and cancer. Basically, he says that "*calcium deficiency in the body fluids outside and inside of the cell stimulates the proliferation of both virus and cell mutation (cancer) by regulating DNA synthesis".* Furthermore, he concludes that *"calcium deficiency is the universal property of all cancer cells, the knowledge of which may be the key to understanding cancer".* He explains that, *"Besides needing calcium ions, normal cells must adequately spread out on a solid substrate before they are able to initiate DNA syntheses. Calcium is specifically required for spreading. Lowering the extra-cellular calcium and preventing spreading both block the initiation of DNA synthesis, without stopping on-going DNA synthesis".* He concludes that *"Calcium must certainly be the major bio-element of the times.*

In other words, calcium is crucial for DNA replication which controls body repair and the maintenance of youth in the body. This explains why some of the cultures around the world, such as the Okinawans who have relatively disease free bodies, also have youthful bodies as they age. In short, *"calcium supplements are the key to the fountain of youth"*.

In addition, to this major activity of calcium, calcium also has another equally important function. When the farmer has acidic soil that won't sustain plant growth, he solves the problem by adding calcium, which wipes out the acid. This ability to wipe out acid is crucial in the human body. Remember that as we get older we drink less and less milk, meaning that our bones slowly become depleted in calcium. This results in the acidification of our body fluids, which unfortunately drives oxygen out of our bodies as oxygen only remains in an alkaline solution and is driven out of acids.

What does this lack of oxygen mean? Well, Dr. Otto Warburg won two Nobel Prizes for proving that cancer was anaerobic or that a lack of oxygen leads to cancer. *Warburg told Dr. Carl Reich that just as water can put out a fire, calcium can wipe the acid out of the human body, resulting in an influx of oxygen.* Other scientists believe that a lack of oxygen can also lead to other degenerative diseases. Therefore, oxygen in the human body is crucial to good health, and calcium with vitamin-D equals oxygen, which is why the longest living cultures all consume huge amounts of calcium and get lots of sunshine. Therefore, America, which is so sick (cancer 40%), is desperate for both calcium and vitamin-D supplementation. The best source of calcium being marine coral calcium from Okinawa, Japan.

CHAPTER SIX

SCIENTIFIC QUOTATIONS

Now that we understand how and why both vitamin-D and calcium work as biological partners, it is time to hear from the scientific medical researchers about their findings.

First some Quotes on Vitamin-D

When we read scientific reports that are several years old, we tend to discredit those reports because they are not modern. Of course this type of reasoning must be considered ridiculous or we would have to disregard the efforts of some of the greatest historical thinkers in modern history. For example, Einstein's theory of relativity was made in the early 1900's, and still is relevant in today's physics. Thus, despite the fact that this tendency to discredit because of age is wrong, a scientific report hot off the press from some of *world's top research scientists* will eliminate this criticism. Therefore, the first quote for vitamin-D comes from a report delivered December 2004 by world renowned cancer oncologists.

But before reading these studies, *the reader must first understand the definition of a telomere and its "Immortal" enzyme, telomerase.* A telomere is a repeated DNA sequence found at the end of chromosomes that protect the chromosome from disintegration. At birth telomeres consist of about 15,000 base pairs of repeated sequences, which become shorter with cell division. Every time a cell divides it loses 25 to 200 DNA base pairs off the telomere ends. Once this pruning has occurred about 100 times the cell ages and does not continue dividing.

What this means is that if the telomere, which protects the ends of all chromosomes, does not break down, then the chromosome will also not break down. This is analogous to a shoe string with a hardened end, where if the hardened end does not fray, then the whole shoestring will remain intact. If this protection occurs, then the shoe string will last forever, just as the cells in the body will last forever and aging can not occur. (Fountain of youth).

The telomere is controlled by its enzyme, "telomerase." Recent research has shown that telomerase activity has been detected in over 85% of over 2000 primary human tumors examined. (*"Vitamin-D: Importance in the Prevention of Cancers, Type 1 Diabetes, Heart Disease, and Osteoporosis", Department of Medicine, Boston University School of Medicine*). Telomerase is present in "Immortal" cancer cells arising from transformation with tumor viral DNA. The telomere shortening in cancer cells is halted by the presence of the enzyme telomerase, which maintains and stabilizes the telomere allowing the cells to divide, or live indefinitely thereby making the cancer cell "immortal". This does not occur in non cancerous cells. Fortunately, as the following clinical studies report, vitamin-D breaks down the telomerase thereby allowing the disintegration of the telomere resulting in a quick death for the once "immortal" cancer cell.

Vitamin-D Clinical Quotes # 1

1) *"Induction of Ovarian Cancer Cell Apoptosis (cell death) by Vitamin-D Through the Down Regulation of Telomerase, The Journal of Biol. Chem., Vol. 279, Issue 51, 5323-53221, December 17, 2004, by Feng Jiang, Junying Bao, Pengfei Li, Santo V. Nicosia, and Weniong Bai, Departments of Pathology and Interdisciplinary Oncology, University of Florida college of Medicine and Programs of Molecular Oncology and Drug Discovery.*

To begin with a telomere is a coating on the end of every cell. As we grow older the telomere gradually shrinks and the cell begins to disintegrate and aging occurs. If the telomere did not shrink, aging would never occur (the fountain of youth). The title of this article is therefore claiming that **vitamin-D degrades cancer telomeres resulting in the death of the cancer.** See quotes:

2) *"Our studies have shown that the growth of cancer is suppressed by vitamin-D"*

3) *"In addition to classic effects on calcium homeostasis, bone density, and mineral metabolism, **the active metabolite***

of vitamin D, modulates cellular proliferation, differ-
rentiation, and apoptosis (the death of the cell) of both
normal and malignant cells."

4)   **"Vitamin-D has been shown to induce apoptosis in**
several human cancer cells, *but little is known about the*
underlying mechanism. **Our study is the first to link the**
down-regulation of (telomerase) due to vitamin-D-induced
apoptosis in cancer cells. "

5)   *"Recent studies from our laboratories have shown that*
the **growth of cancer is suppressed by vitamin-D through**
cell arrest at the telomere"

6)   **"Our data suggests that vitamin-D exerts a long**
lasting effect on cancer cells because the loss of ability to re-
grow correlates with apoptosis (programmed cell death)"

7)   *"Besides decreased growth rate,* **cancer cells lost their**
ability to regrow after the removal of vitamin-D if they had
been treated continuously for longer than 6 days".

8)   *"To become immortal, human cancers are invariably*
associated with activation of a mechanism that maintains
telomere length. **Our study shows that the telomere in cancer**
cells are disintegrated by vitamin-D thereby removing
cancer's immortality."

9   *"It is important to point out that the disintegration of*
telomerase by vitamin-D is detectable in breast cancer
cells."

Vitamin-D Clinical Quotes # 2

" Vitamin D: importance in the prevention of cancers, type 1 diabetes, heart disease, and osteoporosis"
From the Vitamin D, Skin, and Bone Research Laboratory, Section of Endocrinology, Diabetes, and Nutrition, Department of Medicine, Boston University School of Medicine, Boston

1) *"The purpose of this review is to put into perspective the many health benefits of vitamin D and the* **role of vitamin D deficiency in increasing the risk of many common and serious diseases, including some common cancers, type 1 diabetes, cardiovascular disease, and osteoporosis."**

2) *"Numerous epidemiologic studies suggest that* **exposure to sunlight,** *which enhances the production of vitamin D_3 in the skin,* **is important in preventing many chronic diseases.** *"*

3) *"***Vitamin D deficiency is prevalent in infants who** *are solely breastfed and who do not receive vitamin D supplementation and in adults of all ages who have increased skin pigmentation or who* **always wear sun protection or limit their outdoor activities.** *"*

4) *"***Vitamin D deficiency is often misdiagnosed as fibromyalgia.** *"*

5) *"Studies in both human and animal models add strength to the hypothesis that the* **unrecognized epidemic of vitamin D deficiency worldwide is a contributing factor of many chronic debilitating diseases. Greater awareness of the** <u>**insidious consequences of vitamin D deficiency**</u> **is needed.** *"*

6) *"Remarkably, it was **the sun's energy that was called on to promote the photosynthesis of vitamin D$_3$ in the skin of vertebrates that was responsible for enhancing the efficiency of intestinal calcium absorption.**"*

7) *".....any process that either decreases the number of UVB photons entering the epidermis or decreases the amount of 7-dehydrocholesterol in the skin **will result in a significant reduction in or the complete elimination of vitamin D$_3$ production in the skin.**"*

8) *"Sunscreens efficiently absorb UVB radiation and therefore markedly diminish the total number of UVB photons that reach the 7-dehydrocholesterol in the skin's cells. **The proper use of a sunscreen with a sun protection factor of 15 reduces the capacity > 99%.**"*

9) *"**Melanin is a natural sunscreen that evolved to protect humans from blistering solar radiation** as they evolved in equatorial regions of the world. This **skin pigment is an extremely effective sunscreen** with absorption properties from the ultraviolet C (200-280 nm) into the visible range (> 700 nm), and it competes quite well with 7-dehydrocholesterol for UVB photons. Therefore, **people of color who have greater amounts of melanin in their epidermis than do whites are less efficient in producing vitamin D$_3$ than are whites. A person with skin type 5/6** (dark skin, never develops a sunburn) **requires 10-50 times the exposure to sunlight to produce the same amount of vitamin D$_3$ in their skin as does a white person with skin type 2 or 3.**"*

10) *"Because the zenith angle is dependent **on time of day, season of the year, and latitude,** those factors have a dramatic effect on the cutaneous production of vitamin D₃."*

11) **"Below ≈35°,** *the zenith angle is more direct, and therefore **pre-vitamin D₃ synthesis can occur in the skin year-round.** However, **above 35° latitude, the angle of the sun is so oblique during the winter months** that most, if not all, of the UVB photons below 315 nm are absorbed by the ozone layer, thereby **either reducing or completely preventing the production of pre-vitamin D₃ in the skin.** "*

12) *"For example, residents of Boston (42 °N), Edmonton, Canada (52 °N), and Bergen, Norway (61 °N) **cannot produce sufficient quantities of vitamin D₃ in their skin for 4, 5, and 6 mo, respectively.** "*

13) **"We observed that 30%, 42%, and 84% of free-living white, Hispanic, and black elderly were vitamin D deficient** *[25(OH)D < 50 nmol/L] at the end of August in Boston. However, it was recently recognized that **42% of African American women aged 15-49 y throughout the United States were vitamin D deficient** [25(OH)D < 40 nmol/L] at the end of the winter."*

14) **"Obesity is often associated with vitamin D deficiency.** *As a person becomes vitamin D-deficient, there is a decrease in the efficiency of intestinal calcium absorption."*

15) *"As early as 1941, Apperly (37) observed that **people living at higher latitudes, eg, Massachusetts and New Hampshire, had a higher risk of dying of the most common cancers than did people living in the South, eg, Georgia and South Carolina."***

16) *"In the late 1980s and early 1990s, **several invest-igators reported increased risks of dying of colon, prostate, and breast cancer in people living at higher latitudes in both the United States and Europe.**"*

17) *"**Grant_reported that ≥25% of the deaths due to breast cancer in women in Europe could be attributed to the women's lack of UVB from exposure to sunlight.**"*

18) *"**Both men and women are at higher risk of dying of cancer if they have minimum exposure to sunlight.**"*

19) *"One of the most intriguing important and unap-preciated biologic functions of 1,25(OH)$_2$D is its **ability to down-regulate hyperproliferative cell growth. Normal and cancer cells that have a vitamin D receptor often respond to 1,25(OH)$_2$D by decreasing their proliferation and enhancing their maturation.**"*

20) *"**The most common autoimmune diseases,** including type 1 diabetes, **rheumatoid arthritis, and multiple sclerosis,** have all been **successfully prevented in models using mice that were prone to these diseases if they received 1,25(OH)$_2$D$_3$ early in life.**"*

21) *"**When nonobese diabetic mice,** who typically develop type 1 diabetes, **received 1,25(OH)$_2$D$_3$ throughout their life, their risk of developing type 1 diabetes was reduced by 80%........children receiving 2000 IU vitamin D from age 1 y on decreased their risk of getting type 1 diabetes by 80%.**"*

22) *"They observed in a mouse model that **1,25(OH)$_2$D is effective in down-regulating renin and angiotensin and thereby decreasing blood pressure.**"*

23) *"The Institute of Medicine reported in 1997 that **the recommended vitamin D intake was inadequate**.......the new recommendations are totally inadequate, **especially if a** person has no exposure to sunlight."*

24) *"**Exposure to sunlight or a tanning bed will correct vitamin D deficiency** in patients with severe intestinal fat-malabsorption syndrome."*

25) *"**Infants and young children who are vitamin D deficient** may be imprinted for the rest of their lives with increased risks **of type 1 diabetes, multiple sclerosis, rheumatoid arthritis, and many common cancers.***

26) *"**Recently, it has been reported that young adults with vitamin D deficiency were at greater risk of congestive heart failure than were their vitamin D-sufficient counterparts.***

Vitamin-D Clinical Quotes - #3

"Vitamin D: its role and uses in immunology"
Department of Biochemistry, University of Wisconsin-Madison, Madison, Wisconsin 53706, USA; and Department of Nutrition, Pennsylvania State University, University Park, Pennsylvania 16802, USA; The FASEB Journal. *2001;15:2579-2585*

1) *"**The significant role of vitamin D compounds as selective immuno-suppressants** is illustrated by their ability to either prevent or markedly suppress animal models of autoimmune disease."*

2) *"Results show that 1,25-dihydroxyvitamin D_3 can either prevent or markedly suppress experimental autoimmune encephalomyelitis, rheumatoid arthritis, systemic lupus erythematosus, type I diabetes, and inflammatory bowel disease."*

3) *"In almost every case, the action of the vitamin D hormone requires that the animals be maintained on a normal or high calcium diet."*

4) *"The vitamin D hormone stimulates transforming growth factor TGFß-1 and interleukin 4 (IL-4) production, which in turn may suppress inflammatory T cell activity. The results suggest an important role for vitamin D in autoimmune disorders and provide a fertile and interesting area of research that may yield important new therapies".*

5) *"Perhaps the most important was the discovery of the VDR, vitamin-D receptor, in the parathyroid glands and the demonstration that the vitamin D hormone functions through its receptor to suppress the preproparathyroid gene and parathyroid cell proliferation."*

6) *"It became evident, therefore, that T cell-mediated immunity is under modulatory control of 1,25-$(OH)_2D_3$, or vitamin-D"*

7) *".....when similar examinations were followed in the high calcium diet, the vitamin D compounds were effective. Therefore, it became clear that calcium is required for the vitamin D suppression of the autoimmune disease, EAE..... The results, therefore, imply that a high calcium diet is required for the vitamin D hormone to be effective in the treatment of EAE."*

Rheumatoid arthritis *proved to be another example of an autoimmune disorder that can be largely prevented by the administration of the 1-hydroxylated vitamin D compounds, including 1,25-(OH)₂D₃......* **high calcium intakes were not required** *for vitamin D compounds to prevent the lesions.*

8) *"....***systemic lupus erythematosus** *(SLE)...... the severity of the MRL symptoms was also markedly prevented by the administration of 1,25-(OH)₂D₃......... the results illustrate that* **a high calcium background is required for the vitamin D hormone to prevent the development of this autoimmune disorder(SLE) in the MRL mice."**

9) *"The laboratory of Margherita Cantorna has investigated the possible treatment or prevention of* **inflammatory bowel disease** *(IBD) by vitamin D.....***Vitamin D deficiency accelerated the appearance of symptoms and increased the severity** *of IBD in interleukin 10 (IL-10) knockout (KO) mice....This was essentially prevented by the administration of 1,25-(OH)₂D₃, again under conditions of* **high calcium intakes***.*

10) *"......we have investigated the development of* **type I diabetes** *in the non-obese diabetic (NOD) mouse model.....***Vitamin D deficiency markedly accelerated the appearance and increased the incidence of type I diabetes** *in the NOD mice.....Addition to the diet of 1,25-(OH)₂D₃ at 50 ng/day for females and 200 ng/day for males* **prevented the appearance of the diabetic lesions***.....the autoimmune disorder in the NOD mice can be prevented by the administration of 1,25-(OH)₂D₃ if animals are receiving a normal* **to high calcium diet."**

11) *"Another important development has been the use of* ***vitamin D compounds to suppress or prevent transplant rejection.***"

12) *"The sum of these findings in whole animals* ***clearly illustrates that T cell-mediated immunity can be regulated by exogenous administration of 1-hydroxylated vitamin D compounds.***"

13) *"Clearly, we are just beginning to probe the mechanisms whereby vitamin D hormone and its analogs can act as selective immuno-suppressants."*

14) *"Suppression of autoimmune disease requires not only the active form of vitamin D and its analogs, but also adequate or* ***high calcium intakes.***"

Vitamin-D Clinical Quotes - #4

1) **"The Calcium Connection"**, Dr. Cedric Garland and Dr. Frank Garland, **1989**, Foreside, Simon and Shuster Inc.

*"****Low cancer areas were far more frequent in the sun belt.*** (This statement is contrary to the incorrect popular belief that sunshine causes cancer). The northern Us states have twice the cancer rate and the southern states. *What was the significance of sunlight with regard to cancer rates? Sunlight reacts with cholesterol inside and on the surface of the skin to create vitamin-D. Vitamin-D helps the body absorb calcium*

and plays a major role in the body's ability to use the calcium that is available."

2) **"Treatment of Vertebral Osteoporosis"**, by Dr. Meunier in the book **Molecular and Cellular Regulation of Calcium and Phosphate Metabolism, 1990** Alan R. Liss Inc.

*"When calcium and vitamin-D is given in daily doses along with moderate amounts of sodium fluoride to patients with osteoporosis, there is a substantial increase in bone mass and a **significant reduction** in the incidence of further vertebral fractures."*

3) *"Further Studies on Intoxification With Vitamin-D"* by L.E. Streck, M.D., H. Deutch, C.I. Reed, PhD., H.C. Struck, PhD., from the College of Medicine, University of Chicago, which was a study on over 773 humans and 64 dogs that lasted for 9 years concluded that *"both human subjects and dogs generally survive the administration of 20,000 IU of vitamin-D per kilogram of body weight per day for indefinite periods without intoxification".* That is equivalent to 33 milligrams for a 180 pound man per day or *"1, 600,000 IU" of vitamin daily* which is *"4000 times"* the current vitamin-D which our medical authorities recommend.

4) Another study by Garfield Snyder M.D., Willard H. Squires M.D., (New York State Journal of Medicine, May 1, 1940, pp708-719) which used doses of 300,000 IU of vitamin-D or 750 times the RDA concluded that *"we are inclined to agree with the Streck Report that the hazards of toxicity in high doses of vitamin-D have been greatly exaggerated as the degree of clinical improvement has* *been marked and sustained with no serious toxic manifestations encountered."*

5)   In another study entitled ***The Treatment of Arthritis By Activated Vitamin-D***, G. Norris M.D. published in ***Rhematism*** July 1947, pages 56-60,   Dr. Norris concludes that *"vitamin-D in massive dosage is of great value in the treatment of arthritis and that toxic effects are so rare or so temporary as to constitute no obstacle to its use."*

6) *Comparative Therapeutic Value and Toxicity of Various Types of Vitamin-D*, by C. Reynolds, M.D., Louisiana State University)   concluded that "intoxification for short periods *does not result in any permanent injury.*"   And that the toxicity of the massive doses given in this study, was probably due to the chemical impurities in the first vitamins manufactured (a problem that had been since corrected) rather than due to the vitamins themselves, and concluded that their findings were the same as Streck, that ***vitamin-D was "non toxic" in amounts "under 20,000 times the RDA"***, which is 160 milligrams or *8,000,000 IU of vitamin-D daily.*

7)   In the 1940's and 1950's, although the doctors began recommending that their patients consume only trace amounts of vitamins, 400 I.U. of vitamin-D (Milk was fortified with vitamin-D).   Ironically, when it came to making money for the drug companies, they routinely prescribed popular drugs such as ***Dalsol, Deltalin and Drisdol, all of which contained over 50,000 I.U. of vitamin-D***. to be taken daily. Thus the patient was told by the doctor that any more than the 400 IU recommended daily allowance of vitamin-D could be toxic, but it was OK to take drugs containing over *250 times* that amount.

8) Dr. Reinhold Vieth of the Department of Laboratory medicine and Pathology, University of Toronto writes in 2004, *"I am amazed at the lack of evidence supporting the statements about the toxicity of moderate doses of vitamin-D and the literature citations supporting toxicity have been either inappropriate or without substance.*

9) A study by Dr Kassandra Munger, Harvard School of Public Health, published in the January 2004 issue of *Neurology* involving 187, 563 women concludes that *"MS is caused in part by lack of sunlight sufficient to allow the body to make its own vitamin-D"*.

10) In a scientific publication (Clin Lab Med. 2000 Sep; 20 (3):569-90) entitled *"Calcium and Vitamin-D Diagnostics and Therapeutics"* Dr. M.F. Holick states that the vitamin-D level in the body should not fall below 3,200 IU and levels below 2,000 IU are considered serious deficiency states and will *"increase your risk of breast and prostate cancer and autoimmune diseases like MS and rheumatoid arthritis"*. He suggests safe levels between 5,000 IU and 15,000 IU. (Remember that the medical authorities will only approve 400 IU daily, thereby inducing these horrific diseases).

11) A question that John Jacob Cannell, M.D., executive Director of the Vitamin-D Council (year 2005) asks his patients is *"If an otherwise healthy adult tried to kill himself by taking an entire bottle of 250 capsules of 1,000 IU of vitamin-D, what would happen?"* Dr Cannell's response is that *"such a one time dose would be a health benefit for the majority of Americans."*

Quotes on Calcium & Cancer

1) *"Coral Calcium exhibited an inhibitory effect on the growth of cancer cells"*
Yuji Hirota, Ph.D., Takashi Sugisaki, Ph.D., *Medical Preventive Groupa Laboratory, MPG Co., Ltd. 2-41-18 Sumida, Sumida-ku, Tokyo, Japan 131*

2) *"A protective effect of calcium on colorectal cancer, one of the most common malignancies in Western societies, has been supported by results of in vitro animal studies."*
Maria Elena Martenez and Walter C. Willett, *Arizona Cancer Center, University ofr Arizona Health Sciences Center, Tuscon, Arizona. And the Channing Laboratory, Harvard Medical School, Department of Nutrition, Boston Massachusetts, 10/30/97.*

3) *"Adding dietary calcium markedly suppressed the diet induced hyper proliferation of epithelial calls (cancer)."*
Lexun Xue, Martin Lipkin, Harrold Newark, Jiarmin Wang, *Influence of Dietary Calcium on Diet Induced Epithelial Cell Hyperproliferation in Mice, Memorial Sloan-Kettering Cancer Center, Strang Cancer Prevention Center, New York, Cell Biology laboratory Henan Medical University, China.*

4) *"Higher calcium intake is associated with a reduced risk of distal colon cancer"*
Kana Wu, Walter C. Willer, Charles S. Fuchs, Graham A. Colditz and Edward L. Giovannucci, *"Calcium Intake and Risk of Colon Cancer in Women and Men", Department of Nutrition, Harvard School of Public Health, Boston MA, Department of Nutrition and Epidemiology, Harvard School*

of Public Health, Channing Laboratory, Harvard Medical School.

5) "The results of the study show that there may be a significant protective effect of calcium intake from drinking water on the risk of rectal cancer."
Chug Yuh Yang and Hui Fen Chui, *"Calcium in Drinking Water and Risk of Death from Rectal Cancer"*, School of Public Health, Department of Pharmacology, Hsiung Medical College, Taiwan.

6) "Both men and women who died of colorectal cancer had a lower mean calcium intake compared to the rest of the population"
Ingrid Slob, Johannes Lambregts, Alberine Schuit and Frans Kok, *"Calcium Intake and Cancer Mortality in Dutch Civil Servants, Department of Epidemiology and Public Health, Agricultural University, The Netherlands*

7) "Our data suggests that high calcium intake may lower colorectal cancer risk"
Paul Terry, John Baron, Lief Bergkvist, Lars Holmberg, and Alicja Wolk, *"Dietary Calcium and Risk of Colorectal Cancer: A prospective Study in Women"*, Nutrition and Cancer, 43(1), 39-46, Department of Medical Epidemiology, Karolinska Institute, Stockholm, Sweden.

8) "The ability of oral calcium supplementation to suppress rectal epithelial proliferation supports its potential to prevent development of colorectal carcinoma in high risk individuals".
M. Thomas, J Thomson, and R Williamson, *"Oral Calcium Inhibits Rectal Epithelial Proliferation in Familial*

Adenomatous Polyposis" Br. J. Surg, 1993, Vol 80, April, 499-501, Department of Surgery, Royal Medical School, St Marks Hospital, London, England.

9) ***"These inhibitory effects on metabolic factors suggest a preventive effect of dietary calcium on colon carcinogenisis".***
R. Van Der Meer, J Lapre, M. Govers, J Kleibeuker, *"Mechanisms of the Intestinal Effects of milk products on Colon Cancer", Cancer letters 114 (9197) 75-83, Department of Nutrition University Hospital Groningen, The Netherlands.*

10) ***"In human subjects at increased risk for colon cancer, hyper-proliferation of colon epithelial cells was reduced after oral dietary supplementation with calcium".***
Harold Newark, and Martin Lipkin, *Cancer Research (suppl) 52, 2067-2070, April1, 1992, Sloan Kettering Cancer Center, New York, Rutgers University College of Pharmacy, New Jersey.*

11) ***"Recent findings have indicated that dietary calcium can modulate and inhibit colon carcinogenisis".***
Sergio Lamprecht and Martin Lipkin, *"Chemoprevention of colon cancer by Calcium", Strang Cancer Prevention Center, New York,*

Quotes on Calcium & Blood Pressure

1) ***"These data suggest that supplementation of dietary calcium may contribute to a reduction of blood pressure in elderly patients with hypertension".***

Yasuyuki Takagi, Masaaki Fukase, Scoichiro Takata, Tadao Fujimi, and Takuo Fujitta, *"Calcium Treatment of Essential Hypertension in Elderly Patients.", Department of Medicine, Kobe University Scholl of Medicine, Kobe, Japan*

2) *"**Treatment with oral calcium** represents well tolerated non-pharmacologic intervention that **lowers blood pressure in patients with mild to moderate hypertension".***
David McCarron, M.D., Cynthia Morris PhD., *"Blood Pressure Response to Oral Calcium in Persons with Mild to moderate Hypertension", Annals of Internal Medicine, December 1985, Volume 103, Number 6, Published by the American College of Physicians, Portland Oregon.*

3) *"**If calcium intake** of the general population **were to increase to above 1200 mg, the incidence of hypertension in the elderly might be decreased".***
Ihab Hajjar, M.D., Clarence Grim, M.D., Theadore Kotchen, M.D., *"Dietary Calcium Lowers the Age-Related Rise in Blood Pressure in the United States", The NHANES Survey, Division of Geriatrics, Department of Internal Medicine, Palmetto Health Alliance University of South Carolina and the Department of Medicine, Medical College of Wisconsin, Milwaukee, WI.*

4) *"**Conclusion, Dietary calcium is inversely related to systolic blood pressure in young children"***
Matthew Gillman, M.D., Susan Oliveria, MPH, Curtis Ellison, M.D., *"Inverse Association of Dietary Calcium With Systolic Blood Pressure in Young Children", From the Evans section of Preventive Medicine and Epidemiology, Boston School of Medicine, Dr Gillman is the recipient of a Physician Investigator Award, American Heart Association.*

5) *"The results of our investigation show that the high calcium diet blunts the development of high blood pressure and may protect against the development of hypertension".*
Wasswa Semafuko, and David Morris, *"Effect of High Calcium Diet on the Development of High Blood Pressure", Department of Pathology and Laboratory Medicine, The Miriam Hospital Division of Biology and Medicine, Brown University, Providence Rhode Island, USA.*

6) *"Calcium intake has been implicated as being important in the development and treatment of hypertension".*
R. Schieffer, and A. Gairard, *"Blood Pressure Effects of Calcium Intake in Experimental Models of Hypertension", Institut de Recherche contre les Cancers, Hopitaux Universitaires, Strasburg, Faculte de Pharmacie, Universite Louis Pasteur, France.*

7) *"The blood pressure-lowering effect of dietary calcium is associated with blunting of thrombin-induced increase in platelet cytosolic calcium".*
Ramachandra Rao, Youxhen Yan, and Yanyuan Wu., *"Dietary Calcium Reduces Blood Pressure" Calcium Hypertension Research Lab, Charles R Drew University of Medicine and Science, Los Angeles, California.*

8) *"The systolic and diastolic arterial blood pressures of rats fed calcium were significantly lower compared to rats of the other groups".*
N Buassi, *"High Dietary Calcium Decreases Blood Pressure in rats", Department de Ciencias Fisiologicas, Centro de*

Ciencias Biologicas   Universidade Estadual de Londrina, Brasil

9)   "The results of our research indicate that calcium restriction accelerates salt-induced hypertension"
M Nakamura, M.D., H Suzuki, M.D., H Yamakawa, M.D., Y Ohno, M.D.,   T Saruta, M.D.,   *"Calcium Restriction Accelerates Salt-Induced Hypertension",   Department of Internal Medicine, Scholl of Medicine,   University of Tokyo, Japan*

Quotes on Calcium & Kidney Stones

1)   "Two powerful prospective observational studies have suggested that increased dietary calcium reduces the risk of kidney stones".
H. Heller, *"The Role of Calcium in the Prevention of Kidney Stones", University of Texas Southwestern Medical Center at Dallas, Texas. J. Am Coll Nutr, 1999 Oct 18, (5 Suppl):373S-378S.*

2)   "Recent evidence suggests that dietary calcium restriction may actually increase the risk of kidney stones and dietary restriction of calcium should be avoided in patients who have kidney stones".
G. Curhan, M.D.,*"Dietary Calcium and Kidney Stone Formation", Channing Laboratory, Department of Medicine, Brigham and Women's Hospital, Boston, Mass.*

3)   "Dietary calcium intake was inversely associated with the risk of kidney stones"

Gary Curhan, M.D., Walter Willet, M.D., Eric Rimm, Sc.D., and Meir Stampfer, M.D., *"A Prospective Study of Dietary Calcium and the Risk of Kidney Stones"*, *Department of Epidemiology and Nutrition, Harvard School of Public Health, Veterans Affairs Medical Center, Boston Mass*

Quotes on Calcium & Bone Fractures

1) *"In 12 of the 19 studies on bone loss in which calcium intake was controlled, all 12 studies showed that calcium conferred a significant benefit".*
R Henley, *"Calcium and Osteoporosis: How Much is Enough", New England Journal of Medicine, 1993;328: 503-505, Pharmaceutical Information Associates Ltd.*

2) *"The capacity of compensatory mechanisms to provide sufficient calcium to offset daily losses from the body declines with age, hence, increasingly <u>the body tears down bone to access its calcium</u>".*
Robert Heaney, M.D., FACN, *"Calcium Needs of the Elderly to Reduce Fracture Risk", Creighteon University, Osteoporosis Research Center, Omaha, Nebraska, Presented at the 41st Annual Meeting pf the American College of Nutrition at Las Vegas, Nevada, Oct 12, 2000.*

3) *"A preventive effect on the risk of hip fracture may partly be achieved by using calcium supplements for a late prevention in elderly people"*

P Meunier, *"Prevention of Hip Fractures by Correcting Calcium Insufficiencies in Elderly People"*, Dept of Rheumat and Bone Disease Hopital Edouard Herriot, Lyon, France

4) **"In elderly women low calcium absorption and intake increases the risk of hip fracture".**
Kristine Ensrud, M.D., Tu Duong, Jane Cauley, Robert Heaney, M.D., Randi Wolf, PhD., Emily Harris, PhD., Steven Cummings, M.D., *"Low Fractional Calcium Absorption Increase the Risk for Hip Fracture in Women With Low Calcium Intake"*, Study of Osteoporotic Fractures Research Group, Ann Intern Med, 2000;132:345-353.

5) **"Thus, oral calcium supplements prevented a femoral bone mineral density decrease and lowered vertebral fracture rate in the elderly".**
T Chevalley, R Rizzoli, V. Nydegger, D Slosman, C Rapin, Jmichel, H Vasey, and J Bonjour, *Effects of Calcium Supplements on Femoral Bone Mineral Density and Vertebral Fracture Rate in Pateients"*, World Health Organization for Osteoporosis and Bone Diusease, Department of Medicine, University Hospital of Geneva, Switzerland.

Quotes on Calcium & Menstrual Disorders

1) **"Based on available evidence, a strong statement can be made regarding the importance of ensuring calcium intake in all women, particularly those in post-menopause".**

The North American Menopause Society (NAMS), *"The Role of Calcium in Postmenopausal Women: consensus opinion of the North American Menopause Society", Menopause 2001, March 8 (2):84-95.*

2)   *"Calcium supplementation is a simple and effective treatment for premenstrual syndrome".*
Susan Thys-Jacobs, M.D., Silvo Ceccarelli, M.D., Arlene Bierman, M.D., Henry Weisman, M.D., Mary Cohen, M.D., Jose Alivir, DrPH, *"Calcium Supplementation in Premenstrual Syndrome", Department of Medicine Metropolitan Hospital, New York Medical College, New York, Society of General Internal Medicine in Washington, D.C.,*

3)   *"Clinical trials in women with PMS have found that calcium supplementation effectively alleviates the majority of mood an somatic symptoms. "*
Susan Thys-Jacobs, M.D., *"Micronutrients and the Premenstrual Syndrome: The Case for Calcium", Clinical Director, Metabolic Bone Center, St. Lukes Roosevelt Hospital, Columbia University, New York*

Note that because vitamin-D and calcium are biological partners, all of the quotes on calcium concerning cancer and blood pressure etc., implies that the presence of vitamin-D is also a crucial factor due to its ability to increase Calcium absorption.

CHAPTER SEVEN

THE CALCIUM FACTOR

In my earlier book entitled **"The Calcium Factor"**, I present viewpoints and statistics that may not be whole-heartedly embraced by conventional medicine. The clear focus of my earlier book was to highlight the underestimated importance of vitamin-D and calcium for health. No healer would doubt the essential nature of calcium, which is the most abundant mineral in the human body, for health, especially related to its role in signaling biochemical processes in cells, controlling muscle contractions, initiating DNA synthesis, and building bones. However, the general level of calcium intake in the Western diet is much lower in many people than is required for optimal health. Furthermore, there are many other ancillary actions of calcium, such as the critical control of the pH (acidity or alkalinity) of the body fluids. This is demonstrated by the fact that body fluids become more acidic with aging when calcium is lacking in the diet. This results in the expulsion of oxygen which can lead to numerous diseases, such as cancer, according to two-time Nobel Prize winner Otto Warburg, the man who discovered the cause and the cure for cancer over 70 years ago.

I have referred to calcium as the *"King of the Bio-elements"*, where deficiency of this element is invariably associated with a whole host of diseases. Calcium, however, does not act alone in the body. It has to be present in abundance with other minerals and co-factors *(especially magnesium and vitamin-D)*, in order that it can play its pivotal role in health. The *"secrets"* of coral calcium for health become unwrapped as we begin to explore the role of coral minerals in supporting the chemistry of life.

My personal odyssey to define the link between minerals and health was reinforced by knowledge that certain geographical locations in the world had inhabitants who were *strangers to illness* and lived to a ripe, old age. Among these long living people are *Abkasians from Georgia, the Hunzas of Pakistan, the Bamas of China, the Vilcabambas of Ecuador and certain Azerbaijans of Russia.* These small populations seem to shave a common factor that they live at high altitude, and they are all outdoor cultures that get a great deal of sunshine. Living at high elevation means an eco system where melting glacial water has an abundant mineral content. The water looks turbid and white and is known around the world as "Milk of the Mountains". Each quart of Hunza water contains about 17,000 milligrams of calcium (or 17 times the content of a quart of milk), and these people drink several quarts of water each day. Therefore, the common denominator with all these outdoor cultures is that their diet is high in mineral nutrients, especially calcium, which are derived from melting glaciers and snow and their exposure to the sun at high elevations which as previously noted increases the amount of vitamin-D produced in each of these cultures. Many other scientists, such as Dr. Carl Reich and Dr. Joe Wallach of "Dead Doctors Don't Lie" fame, have correctly proposed that these minerals factor in longevity. Despite the outcry of incompetence by the medical authorities, Carl Reich and Joe Wallach were right and they (your current medical authorities) are wrong!!! Carl Reich and Joe Wallach should go down in history as two of the greatest nutritionists of all times. They both deserve medals.

This association between abundant mineral intake, sunshine and health is supported by the finding that sea level populations with health and longevity, such as the Okinawans in Japan, have a similar abundance of minerals in their diet and sunshine in their lives. In the case of the Okinawans, their source of Calcium is from the coral reefs around the Rukuyuku islands. These reefs provide mineral calcium enrichment to the water supply and coral to the ocean floor which is often taken as a supplement in the diet, or mixed with their food preparations. Again, the *"experts"* will claim that it is only an *"interesting"* coincidence, preferring to believe that it is good food and a sedentary lifestyle, but the shear number of coincidences of high calcium intake with sunshine, after a while, start to *imply* real proof of the cause and effect. The key to good health and longevity is therefore *"calcium and sunshine"*.

While minerals may not be the whole story of health and longevity, they definitely are much more important than has been previously supposed. Unfortunately, there has been a tendency in modern medicine to reject remedies of natural origin, such as coral, that have centuries of precedence of successful use. Modern medicine definitely rejects the sun as a good source of nutrition, with all doctors screaming that it causes cancer. But fortunately, the pendulum is now swinging in the opposite direction as pluralistic medicine emerges and we move back to basics in applying optimum lifestyle and nutrition for health. Also, the information exchange of the internet is having a huge impact. In addition, books like the one you are reading are opening the eyes of many. Coral Calcium serves as an historical example of a natural agent from the ancient seas which holds great power for health and well-being. Vitamin-D is in the same category.

It is also unfortunate that doctors are also incorrectly screaming that cholesterol causes heart disease. Heart disease is the number one killer in North America, with cancer a close second. Important facts about cholesterol are that it is a vital component of the body, it is found in every cell, it is a component of steroid hormones such as testosterone and estrogen. It is used to conduct nerve impulses, and it is present in large quantities in the brain (70%) and bile. Additionally, cholesterol is one of the constituents of the skin that is *crucial to the production of sun-on-skin vitamin-D*. Finally, but not least important, about 80% of all body cholesterol is not ingested in the diets, but rather, is manufactured by the body. In the April 1997 issue of the *New England Journal of Medicine,* Kilmer McCully M.D. reports a radical *"new"* medical theory that cholesterol *"is not the primary cause"* of heart disease, but rather, *"acid causing the inflammation of blood vessel walls"* is the primary cause of heart attacks and strokes". The resulting debris, caused by the acidosis degeneration, along with fibrin phospholipids, collagen and cholesterol, creates a patch to repair the break. Goopy cholesterol binds everything together. Therefore cholesterol is not only one of the most biologically important molecules in the body, but it is also involved in repairing the body not in damaging the body. Thus, all cholesterol drugs disrupt this natural biological process & cause death. (ie: Vioxx)

CHAPTER EIGHT

OKINAWA AND CORAL CALCIUM

The library of Congress in Washington DC has over 17,000 scientific publications on calcium and disease. There are literally thousands of quotes from the world's best medical researchers claiming that calcium can both prevent and reverse disease. It is interesting to note that no researcher will ever use the word *"cure"* for fear of loosing all of his research funding, but there message is clear. They use every word but the word *"cure"*. One inventive cancer researcher writes that the calcium makes the diseased cancer cells *"grow back to normal"*. There are also many scientists reporting that vitamin-D also helps to inhibit and reverse cancer. Therefore, calcium, working hand in hand with vitamin-D *"cure's* cancer and a host of other diseases. It is Bob Barefoot's opinion (and remember that Barefoot has been studying biological calcium almost longer that any of today's scientists and is known today by many as The King of Calcium) that the best form of nutrient calcium is *"marine coral calcium"* from Okinawa Japan, to which this chapter is devoted.

Okinawa, composed of hundreds of coral reef islands, is located at the southern tip of the mainland of Japan. Some of the islands were created by volcanic activity which filled the waters around the islands with mineral nutrients for the coral to absorb. It is a Prefecture (Province) with approximately one and one half million inhabitants. Native Okinawans are among the healthiest and are the longest living people in the world. Recent population statistics show that Okinawa has more centenarians than other parts of Japan, and ten times as many per capita as the United States. Japan itself is noted for longevity, but Okinawa stands out as a special location for health, well-being and elite elderly inhabitants. The average number of people at or over the age of 100 years is *29 per 100.000* of the population compared with the national, Japanese average of *9 per 100.000* people. This compares with about *3 per 100,000* of the population in the United States or almost a ten fold difference. In the late 1990's approximately 400 people in Okinawa were recorded to be living beyond their 100th birthday, and those in their 80's and 90's lead extremely robust, active, healthy, youthful and productive lives, the same as Americans in their 20's or 30's. This longevity among Okinawans is striking.

It is recorded in folklore and legends that an Emperor of China sent a mission of three thousand explorers to find the land of *"heaven on earth"*. This heavenly place was called *"Horai"* - according to legend – and it was believed to be present in the warm ocean off the east coast of China. The Chinese Emperor was seeking the elixir of life (or *"fountain of youth"*) and he commanded his missionaries to bring him back the life sustaining tonic. To the Emperor's dismay, the mission did not return. Legend states that these Chinese explorers found an island paradise that was too satisfying for

74

them to leave. This island was considered the land mass of *"eternal life"*. Legend identifies this place as the prefecture of Okinawa, with its coral base and pristine, clear seas.

Many cultures hold similar legends, but the quality and length of life of the inhabitants of Okinawa make this story plausible. Understanding how the habitat of Okinawa promotes health and well-being has been a key focus of anti-aging research for several decades. Whilst one should not believe in *"fairy tales"*, modern researchers have increasingly found that folklore is a great starting point to examine new scientific concepts in natural medicine. In fact, researchers at the National Institutes of Health in the US have used folklore accounts of remedies of natural origin to select botanicals and marine organisms for investigation and research as new treatments. This approach has been found to be especially valuable and productive in the search for new anti-cancer compounds.   Perhaps this is why Okinawan folklore for thousands of years has taught that *"the islands of Okinawa shall one day cure the world."*

Okinawan people view food and medicine as synonymous.   This was also the view of the Father of Medicine, Dr. Hippocrates, who declared 2500 years ago that *"All food was medicine and the best food was the best medicine"*.   This inseparability of food from medicine is a foreign concept to the Food and Drug Administration (FDA) who continue to ignore the medicinal qualities of food while extolling the virtues of killer drugs. Also, this inseparability of food from medicine is reflected in the phrase *"Nuchi-Gusui"* which is used in Okinawa to give thanks for food. In contrast, the term *"Gochi-Soo-Sama"* is a common phrase for giving thanks for meals in mainland Japan. When roughly translated the term *"Nuchi-Gusui"* used by the Okinawans means *"The Life Medicine"*. This cultural attitude to food which emphases the act eating to support body structure and function is absent in many Western societies, especially the United States with its horrific track record of disease. Certainly, this attitude is also inconsistent with the American *"Double Whopper Brain"* and **Big Gulp Society"** that has created many other *"Fast Food Nations"*.

The most popular staple in the diet of Okinawans is *"firm tofu"* which is used with calcium in its preparation. The act of *"**adding coral calcium"*** to tofu has been variably practiced by Okinawans and ensures optimal mineral intake

Recorded in the history of Okinawa is the phenom-enon of exodus of physicians. Local folklore history holds that physicians and healers left Okinawa when coral was included increasingly in the diet of the local populations. This circumstance was attributed to a precipitous decline in disease which tended to make the physicians redundant. This lack of doctors was noted by the Spanish explorers who believed correctly that the reason was coral calcium, and thus they filled their ship holds with coral calcium instead of the customary gold bullion. In addition, popular history refers to **enhanced agricultural production** when coral was used in agricultural practices as fertilizer and a food supplement. It should be noted that the Okinawans were a highly educated society that they meticulously documented their history, and therefore the stories are much more than simply hearsay. Besides this, it is well known that the secrets of life are derived from the oceans.

While we are still exploring the landmass of the earth, the oceans hold many secrets that are relatively inaccessible. This under-explored frontier of waters of the worlds' surface has a volume of 42 million billion cubic ft or 286 million cubic miles. Experts believe, for instance, that the average gold content is 0.012 parts per billion. This calculates out to be *460,000,000,000 ounces of gold* or over 100 times the gold currently held in the world's vaults. Thus, the oceans are an enormous collection of metals, minerals and chemical substances that sustain life and that can be absorbed by the coral. The seas contain many factors that are produced by its' own living organisms.

The sea is also rich in salt (sodium chloride) and every natural element known to man is present at one or another location. The contents of the sea are determined to a major degree by its residents, but oceans have many citizens who live in different geographic locations with distinct climates. It therefore appears that diverse ecology in the seas mirrors the diversity of life that is encountered on landmasses of the earth.

The chemical balance in the oceans supports life in complex ways. Therefore, one cannot be surprised by scientific reports that many marine life forms and their environmental waters or habitants, such as coral reefs, produce substances that have potent and versatile biological actions in nature. Marine compounds of various types have been found to be antifungal, antibiotic, anticancer, antiviral, growth inhibiting, analgesic, cardio-stimulatory (or inhibitory) in their actions.

To add to our appreciation of the health secrets that the oceans contain is the recognition that four fifths of all life on our planet (about one half million species) lives in water. Massive amounts of suspended organic matter are incorporated into the food chain of marine organisms. Furthermore, marine organisms, such as living corals or mussels, process or expose their life cycle to thousands of tons of water. In one estimate, a small colony of mussels (ten million) can process one square mile of sea water that is 25' deep. As *"big fish eats little fish"* or marine organisms are used in complex food chains, the permutations of transfer of active molecules becomes limitless. Humankind joins this complex harmony of planetary life when it harvests the offerings of the oceans, such s coral calcium.

Bacteria and primitive life forms that thrive in and around these underwater vents have basic *"genetic material"* that suggests that they are related to all organisms on the earth. In other words, the genetic material or nucleic acid (RNA) found in these organisms is similar to that in all animal life. This finding has led to new proposals about the origin of life on earth. It has been proposed that life developed in warm sea waters, perhaps around these submersed vents. Life is believed to have begun in the seas about 3.3 billion years ago and studies of deep sea communities regularly *"turn up"* new species of organisms.

Many drugs and nutrients have been derived from marine sources, but the health secrets of the oceans remain sadly under-explored. For examples, marine sources of omega 3 fatty acids are essential nutrients that have wide ranging health benefits including the promotion of cardiovascular health, immune function and optimal structure and function of the central nervous system. Extracts of coral have been shown to have antibacterial and anti-inflammatory properties, in addition to the value of coral calcium as a mineral source.

Corals belong to the phylum (group) of marine organisms called Cnidaria (Coelenterata) which also includes jellyfish, sea anemones and hydroids. These organisms tend to be symmetrical with a digestive tract that has one single opening. They possess a *"nematocyst"* or stinging apparatus which contains and protects the coral polyp with venom of varying potency. The stony corals are named because they secrete a supporting exoskeleton (outside hard structure). This stony covering contains the soft structures of the living coral polyps. These living corals form reefs which support a large biomass. Coral reefs yearly secrete clouds of sperm to flood and impregnate the reefs to create new growth. In tropical waters and some temperate zones these corals proliferate to a vast degree that builds islands. A classic example of this geographic phenomenon is the infrastructure of the island chains in and around Okinawa, Japan.

Coral calcium is derived from reef-building coral and it is harvested from the pristine waters in deep ocean troughs many miles off the Nansei Islands (Rukuyuku and Satsunan), Japan.. These islands spread towards the south east from the southern tip of Japan's main land mass towards Taiwan. The coral that is broken off by wave action or munching fish (coral calcium) is carried by ocean currents miles out into the ocean where it is deposited in deep sea troughs and can be harvested without disturbing the reefs. Using careful, harvesting techniques that are sustaining for the environment, several companies collect and process coral calcium for use as a food supplement. The Japanese government supervises this collection process and they provide special certification to certain types of coral.

Therefore, any criticism that the reefs are endangered is totally absurd as the coral, which is harvested ecologically safe, is not even harvested from the reefs. It is important to recognize that two broad, but distinct types of coral calcium are used as health giving supplements by the Japanese and many people throughout the world. The first type is fossilized calcium that has been deposited on the land mass, or washed up on to beaches. The second type is taken directly from the sea bed. The sea-bed coral is the coral that has dropped from the reef or is processed by reef inhabitants. This type of *"coral sand"*, marine coral, has been washed to the ocean floor by wave actions. Marine coral is closer in composition to the living forms of corals, because the marine microbes are still active and many minerals and organic elements are retained, in comparison to fossilized, land-based coral, which by environmental activity, such as storms, have had much of the mineral nutrients washed out. Unscrupulous companies selling the cheap and inferior fossilized coral spread the fear that the reefs are being damaged so that people will refrain from buying the high grade marine coral, and purchase their dirt cheap dirt coral instead.

Under a microscope, coral appears as tubes, horns and honey combs. It has the appearance of a fascinating and abandoned ancient city. Coral calcium has been officially recognized by the Japanese government as a valuable food supplement. This official standing was registered by Japan in

July 1989, but the coral sands have enjoyed thousands of years of local use as an important source of health giving nutrients in the diet of Okinawans. It was discovered by the early Spanish explorers, over 500 years ago, who filled their ship holds with the coral sands, instead of the usual gold bullion. The chemists in Spain, attempting to discover the reason for its miraculous curative properties, discovered that the main ingredient was calcium, so the coral sands were re-named *"coral calcium"*. Today, tens of millions of people around the world consume coral calcium daily.

There are important differences in composition between fossilized (land-based) coral and marine (sea-bed) coral. Marine coral contains more magnesium, and the balance of calcium (24%) to magnesium (12%) content of this second type of marine coral is close to 2 to 1. This 2 to 1 ratio, according to many biochemists, is the ideal ratio for calcium and magnesium intake in the human diet. Barefoot's research has led him to believe that the natural, magnesium enriched, marine coral is to be strongly preferred as a health giving supplement over land based (fossilized coral), which contains less than 1% magnesium. This superiority is due to its retained, ideal, ionic balance of calcium and magnesium in a 2:1 ratio, and the fact that a host of other nutrients were also washed out during weathering processes.

Before we explore the chemical composition of coral and its nutritional content, its origin and complexities of development must be appreciated. Coral polyps are clever builders of underwater domains that are teaming with plant and animal life. Of major interest is the observation of longevity and health of the inhabitants of the reef islands of Okinawa, Japan. These islands are a source of coral calcium that has a long recorded history of use as a health-giving food supplement. It is interesting to note that coral from other locations around the world does not have the same health benefits. Okinawan coral is unique in that the coral of Okinawa is constantly being fed volcanic nutrients and the marine microbes contained are found only in Okinawa. Also it is unique in that the coral calcium is collected in deep ocean troughs, miles from the reefs, where for millions of years it continues to collect and absorb nutrients from the ocean. Because of this, there is enough marine coral from Okinawa to cure the world many times over.

CHAPTER NINE

VITAMIN-D TOXICITY

Almost every American doctor has the opinion that "vitamin-D can be toxic". There are absolutely no scientific studies that support this theory. Dr. Reinhold Vieth of the Department of Laboratory Medicine and Pathology, University of Toronto writes, *"I am amazed at the lack of evidence supporting the statements about the toxicity of moderate doses of vitamin-D and the literature citations supporting toxicity have been either inappropriate or without substance.* In order to dispel the myth of vitamin-D toxicity, an examination of scientific studies will demonstrate that Dr. Veith is correct when he said that they are either inappropriate or without substance. Dr Veith in the 1999 issue of the American Journal of Clinical Nutrition writes that the minimum effective amount of vitamin-D is *4000 IU* daily or 10 times the current RDA. He says that there are no adverse effects under *10,000 IU* daily which he recommends. He is joined by Dr. Joseph Mercola, who recommends similar amounts to help prevent breast cancer. Also, according to the Harvard School of Public Health there is a significant association between vitamin-D deficiency and prostate cancer risk.   Dr. Jonathan V. Wright points out in his "Nutrition and Healing" newsletter that *"sun exposure is not only good for you, it's essential"*.

The January 13, 2004 edition of the Arizona Republic in an article entitled "Vitamin-D Addition May Lower Risk of MS" writes that in a study involving 187,563 women that *"MS may be caused in part by a lack of sunlight sufficient to allow the body to make its own vitamin-D"*. And another large North American study found that *"higher vitamin-D levels appear to give significant protection against cancer of the colon"*. The researchers found that the group with the lowest vitamin-D intake was 2.5 times more likely to develop bowel cancer than those with the most vitamin-D in their diet.

Laboratory studies have found that there are receptor sites for vitamin-D on cancer cells, and it appears capable of converting human leukemia cancer cells back into normal healthy cells. And finally, the February 2, 2005 edition of the Arizona Republic in an article entitled, *"Sunlight Emerges as a Cancer Risk Remedy"* reports that new research indicates that *"sunlight may help victims survive melanoma"*. Having shown all these positive studies, doctors, who are obviously in a state of denial, will still speculate that vitamin-D is toxic and will claim, incorrectly, that there must be studies to prove it.   Dr. Carl Taylor, a medical pioneer from Edmonton, Canada reports that the medical community is constantly being bombarded by the medical authorities and drug industry with technical information *"suggesting that vitamin-D was toxic"*

But, before we examine the vitamin-D studies, it is important to understand the history of vitamin-D. I learned of its potency when in 1982, Dr Carl Reich, M.D. showed me the autopsies on several terminal cancer patients that he had treated with large doses *"vitamin-D and calcium"*. None of the autopsies showed any cancer. Thus, I concluded that Dr. Reich had indeed *"cured cancer"* in many of his patients. Dr. Reich explained to me that back in the late nineteen twenties people were taking what was called megavitamins and the hospitals were virtually empty. Hospitals had a medical emergency as they were losing money and had to fill the hospital beds. At about this time, a study on vitamin-D was performed where seven medical students were given massive doses of vitamin-D, enough to kill a horse. Vitamin-D was then quickly removed from the market following the toxic effects that these massive doses had on these medical students.

The American public demanded the government intervene and conduct a fair study of whether vitamin-D was toxic. Many people had commonly taken what was known as *"mega doses"*, for example 20 milligrams of vitamin-D for a woman, who would then claim dramatic health benefits, including empty hospitals. The government concurred with the people and gave the job of determining whether vitamin-D was toxic to the prestigious *University of Chicago medical facility*. The study spared no expense and using large numbers of people and animals, required hundreds of doctors and scientists. This study took nine years to complete. The results were as follows:

85

Study #1. --- *Further Studies on Intoxification With Vitamin-D* --- I.E. Streck, M.D., H. Deutsch, A.B., C.I. Reed, PhD., H.C. Struck, PhD., College of Medicine, University of Illinois, Chicago, **Annuals of Internal Medicine**, Volume 10, Number 7, **January 1937**. (9 year study on 64 dogs and 773 people). With the following quotes:

1) *"Early experience with **impure preparations of vitamin-D** has lead to a great deal of **misunderstanding** and fear of over-dosage on the part of those who have little acquaintance with the fundamental mechanisms involved. Suffice it to say that **most of the earlier work must be disregarded.** "*

2) *"With eight exceptions, all of the 43 dogs receiving more than 20,000 I. U. per day per kilogram of body weight died spontaneously. "* *(between 8 and 120 days and an average of over 26 days).* **Note:** *this minimum dosage was equivalent to **14,545,000 I.U for a 160 pound man** which is over **36,000 times** the current RDA. The maximum dosage was 500,000 I.U per kg or over 36,000,000 I.U. for a 160 pound man which is over **90,000 times** the current RDA,"* **which is enough to kill a horse.**

3) *"Among the 20 dogs receiving the lower dose, 20,000 units/kilogram **(equivalent to 14,545,000 I.U. for a 160 pound man or 36,000 times the current RDA,)**, there was **"no evidence of cell injury"**, insignificant weight loss, very little evidence of toxic symptoms, and with the exception of two dogs that died from distemper, **all were in good condition."***

4) *"From these experiments it appears that "dogs may recover from extreme stages of toxicity and that whatever tissue injury occurs may be repairable."*

5) *"There were **"no deaths"** among the 773 human subjects whose doses routinely given ranged upward from 200,000 I.U. total daily dose (**500 times the RDA**) for periods ranging **from seven days to five years**. "*

6) *"One of the authors took 3,000,000 I.U. total daily (**7,500 times the current RDA**) for 15 days **without any evidence of disturbance of any kind**. "*

7) *"Both human subjects and dogs generally **"survive"** the administration of 20,000 I.U. per kilogram (or the 1,800,000 I.U equivalent for a 180 pound man or **4,500 times** the RDA) per day **for indefinite periods without intoxification**. "*

8) ***"Intoxification for short periods does not result in any permanent injury** that can be recognized by the methods employed in this investigation ".*

9) *"In view of the extensive experience in administration of vitamin-D to human subjects with a relatively low incidence of toxicity, and the correlation of the results of animal experiments with the observations on human subjects, we believe that "**the burden of proof now rests on those who maintain the undesirability of the use of this form (high daily doses of vitamin-D) of therapy**."*

Shortly after this massive study (which found large dosages of vitamin-D to be both ***non-toxic*** and ***beneficial to health***, and which was ignored by the American Medical Association) was concluded, the drug companies responded by introducing a new class of **drugs**, such as **Dalsol, Deltalin, and Drisdol**. These drugs were nothing more than vitamin-D (over 50,000 I.U) with a filler. These expensive drugs made from inexpensive vitamin-D were so effective that the deceived public were so impressed with these *"new drugs"* developed by the drug industry that they did not mind paying a high price for something that finally worked. Dr Riech says that the drug industry was not doing well in the late 1930's with the beginning of World War II, but the vitamin-D drugs helped to save the drug industry. Therefore, the drug industry has personal experience as to the effectiveness of vitamin-D in stopping disease in its tracks, even though they publicly claim that *"vitamin-D may be toxic"*.

While the Streck study was still underway, the medical authorities undertook another major initiative, to deceive the public. In order to sway people from taking large doses vitamins which they knew would cure them; they had to find a way to make people think that they were taking *"too much"*. First they began with the propaganda that vitamin *"may be toxic"* or *"could be toxic"*. Then they used reverse psychology to trick the public. They took the more crucial vitamins, vitamin-D, vitamin-E and vitamin-A, and changed their units of measurement. Prior to this everything was measured in milligrams. For example, *most women were taking 20 milligrams of vitamin-D,* which was 1/3rd the 60 milligrams of vitamin-C they would get from eating an Orange. The new units were called **"International Units or IU's"** and the 20 milligrams of vitamin-D became 1,000,000 international units (IU's), which sounds like it is way too much to take. After all, the woman eating the orange was only getting 60 milligrams of vitamin-C, how could she ever take 1,000,000 vitamin-D. So the average woman would take 400 IU of vitamin-D along with 60 mg of vitamin-C that she could get from eating an orange. The numbers to this day sound reasonable, even though they are ridiculous. The reverse psychology or numbers psychology worked and appears to be even more effective today. The problem is that even though the numbers sound reasonable, *the reality is that the woman is now getting less than one one-hundredth of one milligram of vitamin-D, thereby guaranteeing that disease would proliferate.* Thus the AMA and FDA coalition had found a way to set the recommended daily allowances (RDA's) so low that disease would become *locked in* which in turn guarantees exorbitant profiteering by the drug industry and medical authorities. *These actions have caused the pain and deaths of millions of Americans.* (25,000,000 from cancer alone since Otto Warburg issued his warning in 1966) Unfortunately, today's doctors are oblivious to these facts, and continue to only prescribe toxic drugs to their patients, with the support of the profiteering drug industry. Appropriately, Dr Carl Reich referred to the RDA's as the *"Recommended Death Amount"* because the values were so low that death would surely occur. In the studies to follow you will see that the 20 milligram level (1,000,000 IU) for vitamin-D is not excessive, but rather it is considered an acceptable dose by medical researchers.

Study #2. --- *Effect of Massive Doses of Vitamin-D on Calcium and Phosphorus Metabolism* --- Karl P. Klassen, M.D., George M. Curtis, M.D., *Archives of Internal Medicine*, Ohio State University College of Medicine, **1939**. With the following quotes:

1) An adequate intake of vitamin-D *is essential* for the optimal utilization of calcium and phosphorus in the normal metabolism of the human body. "

2)   During four three-day periods, vitamin-D was given beginning with a dose of 200,000 I.U. per day. This was increased by 200,000 I.U. during each of the two succeeding three day periods. During the last period, each patient received 1,000,000 I.U. per day (**2,500 times** *the current RDA*). **None** of the patients showed signs of toxicity. During the last three days there ensued an increase in appetite and the patients had less discomfort. There was neither loss of weight nor marked change in the clinical picture. The blood pressure remained normal."

Note that this study found that giving over *500 times* to *2,500 times* the RDA, *" vitamin-D, was not toxic".*

Study# 3. --- *A Preliminary Report on Activated Ergosterol --- (A form of High Dosage Vitamin-D in the Treatment of Chronic Arthritis),* G. Garfield Snyder, M.D., F.A.C.P., Willard H. Squires, M.D., F.A.C.P., *New York State Journal of Medicine,* **May 1, 1940**, pp 708-719. With the following quotes:

1)   We started our (four year) experiment by giving only 50,000 I.U. a day. This dosage was gradually increased. Finally *we came to the conclusion that it is fairly* safe *to start a dose of 150,000 I. U. a day (*375 times *the RDA)*. During the past two years we have increased our dosage from 100,000 I.U.to a general average of 300,000 I.U. (**750 times** *the current RDA*) In some instances we have gone as high as 500,000 and 600,000 I.U. In most cases this average dose of 300,000 I.U. was maintained throughout the entire period of treatment. "

"We are inclined to agree with Reed, Struck and Streck that *the hazards of toxicity in high dose vitamin-D therapy have been greatly exaggerated."*

2) The question of relative degree of toxicity of the various vitamin-D preparations in the treatment of chronic arthritis assumes great importance in the final determination of the value of high-dosage vitamin-D. The *original technique* of irradiation of ergosterol (vitamin-D), followed by extraction of vitamin-D by means of alcohol, *was not designed* to obtain a product intended *for massive doses*. With the *new Whittier method*, the ergosterol is brought to a boil and the vapor is subjected to the activating influence of an electric current. This vapor is subsequently conducted off and crystallized. The manufacturer *claims that ergosterol manufactured in this manner will prove nontoxic if used in massive doses for the treatment of arthritis. "*

3) "The results indicate that the administration of vitamin-D, prepared by the Whittier method, in the high dosage of this study benefited the great majority of these patients in varying degrees. In a relatively high percentage of cases, *the degree of clinical improvement has been marked and sustained. No serious toxic manifestations were encountered. "*

Once again, a sustained study, four years, of consuming levels of vitamin-D up to *1,500 times* the RDA, was both *"non-toxic and beneficial to health"*, and that the hazards of vitamin-D had been *"greatly exaggerated"*.

Study #4. --- *Follow-up Study of Arthritic Patients Treated with Activated Vaporized Sterol* --- R. Garfield Snyder, M.D., F.A.C.P., Willard H. Squires, M.D., F.A.C.P., *New York State Journal of Medicine,* December, 1941. With the following quotes:

1) There is no consistent change in the Blood calcium. "

2) Most of the cases showed an increase in weight. One of the early signs of activated vitamin-D administration is a *markedly improved* sense of well-being and a definite improvement in nutrition".

" We believe that *"the use of high doses of activated vitamin-D is not associated with any more danger than is usually encountered with other accepted forms of therapy".*

O nce again, high doses of the activated vitamin-D were found to be *non-toxic*.

Study #5. --- *Comparative Therapeutic Value and Toxicity of Various Types of Vitamin-D* --- Chapman Reynolds, M. D. , Louisiana State University School of Medicine, *The Journal Lancet,* Minneapolis, **October, 1942**, Vol LXII, No. 10, page 372. With the following quotes:

1) It may be concluded beyond little doubt that *"massive doses"*, quantities *exceeding by a thousand times* or more the minimal requirement (note this is not the current RDA of 400 I.U., but rather the minimum requirement of 10,000 I.U required to treat arthritis), of *irradiated ergosterol,*

manufactured in Germany in the late 1920s and early 1930s, may result in considerable impairment of nutrition, loss of weight, pronounced hypercalcemia, and abnormal calcium deposits in certain tissues and organs. There are contrasting expressions from users of the electrically stimulated ergosterol (Whittier process), which reported *"favorable results with no toxic reactions"* and the serum calcium not elevated above the normal. "

2) A study of the administration of vitamin-D leads to the belief that contradictory findings indicate that various workers were using different types of preparations. It is strikingly evident that massive doses of irradiated ergosterol bring about the development of toxic effects without clinical improvement, while use of electrical-discharge activated heat-vaporized ergosterol (Whittier process) has consistently been followed by clinical improvement with frequent rehabilitation, and with negligible or *"no toxic manifestations even over prolonged periods of intensive treatment"*.

Thus, study#5 shows that the original toxic effects that resulted from taking thousands of times the minimal requirement (over 250,000 times the current RDA), were not caused by the vitamin-D, but were caused by *"the impurities of using the solvent extracted and irradiated procedure to produce the vitamin-D."* This only occurred in the initial years of the manufacture of vitamin-D. It also concluded that the same amounts of the newer and cleaner form of vitamin-D produced by the new Whittier process was both *non-toxic and beneficial to health*. The suggestion that vitamin-D could result in illness was caused by a misconception and a total lack of understanding, which continues to this day, by our medical authorities.

This was not the first time, as *these same medical authorities also told the world that vitamin-A,* which they believed to be highly beneficial to human health, *caused the deaths of our early arctic explorers*, as they loved to eat polar bear livers which contained 8,000,000 I.U.'s. This propaganda was effective at swaying people from taking vitamin-A. Documents of the day however, dispute this claim, as no explorer died. They do however claim that the explorers suffered from hair loss and dermatitis. Then, in 1983 a team of *Swedish scientists studying the arctic waters discovered that the seal and polar bear livers were collecting and concentrating cadmium found in the water.* The hair loss and dermatitis of the early explorers were caused by cadmium poisoning and not the vitamin-A. Once again the drug industry prevails with propaganda and misinformation.

Study #6. --- *The Therapeutic Value of Electrically Activated Vaporized Ergosterol (Vitamin-D)* --- Cornelius H. Traeger, M.D. F.A.C.P., Willard H. Squires, M.D., F.A.C.P., Emmanuel Rudd, M.D., Arthritis Clinic Hospital for Special Surgery, New York City, *Industrial Medicine*, 14:3, March 1945. With the following quotes:

1) Electrically activated vaporized ergosterol treatment given once weekly in doses of 1,000,000 to 1,500,000 I.U **(3,750 times *the current RDA*)** proved beneficial in the majority of the patients treated. "

2)   *The safety* of electrically activated vaporized ergosterol (Whittier process) when administered orally *has been established* and its effectiveness as an anti-arthritic means of therapy has been repeatedly shown.   The previous findings have been confirmed and extended. "

Once again, the *"effectiveness and safety"* of the vitamin-D produced by the Whittier process was proven.

Study #7.   ---   *The treatment of Arthritis By Electrically Activated Vaporized Ergosterol,*   ---   G. Norris, M.D., *Rheumatism,* **July 1947,**   pages 56-60. With the following quotes:

1)   For vitamin-D produced by the electrically activated vaporized process it is widely claimed that *"in massive dosage it is of great value in the treatment of arthritis"*, and that *"toxic effects are so rare or so temporary as to constitute no obstacle to its use"*.   In a series of 164 cases treated at Cook County Hospital the blood-calcium level was determined before vitamin-D therapy was started, and then at six-month intervals: *"no persistent hypercalcemia developed"*

2)   A clinical trial has been started with a series of 40 patients. After 6-12 months (50,000 to 300,000 I.U. per day), a survey gives the following results:

> Reduction in pain joints, 23 patients (58%)
> Reduction in swelling & stiffness in joints...
> 18 patients (45%)
> General improvement (feeling splendid)......
> 31 patients (78%)

Of evidence of toxicity, the only ones observed were gastric disturbances in 16 of the 40 patients which ranged from a feeling of *"fullness"* or *"a lump"* in the stomach through varying degrees of "feeling of sickness" with the bigger doses.

Once again, the *"effectiveness and safety"* of the vitamin-D produced by the Whittier process was proven. Also, although no persistent hypercalcemia developed, it is interesting to note that massive Japanese studies have found that although large amounts of some calcium nutrients have been associated with hypercalcemia, no amount of coral calcium has ever caused the problem. One also wonders with all of this evidence, what do the negative studies say. Well, the next study is a perfect example of a flawed evaluation.

Study #8. --- *Intoxification With Vitamin-D* --- John Eager Howard, M.D. and Richard J. Meyer, M.D., John Hopkins Hospital, Baltimore, *The Journal of Clinical Endocrinology,* Volume 8, Number 11, November 1948. With the following quotes:

1) The age of the 10 patients given the drug (vitamin-D) as a therapeutic measure against arthritis varied from 33 to 68 years. The highest daily dose was *600,000 I.U*; the lowest daily dose was *150,000 I.U.* (each patient received one of four different drugs, and one patient received a combination of two different drugs). Duration of therapy prior to the onset of toxic symptoms was highly variable, ranging from two months to eighteen months. One patient received a quart

of milk daily and another had been given calcium phosphate wafers coinciding with vitamin-D therapy. "

2)   Eight of the ten patients had severe gastro-intestinal symptoms, namely, anorexia, nausea and vomiting. Weakness, fatigue and lassitude were prominent complaints of all ten.   All our patients were given *diets very low in calcium* on recognition of their condition: yet hypercalcemia was slow to regress.   It seems likely that the bones were the major source of the excess calcium in the serum.

3)..Seven of the ten arthritic patients *"insisted that their joint symptoms were improved"* during the period of vitamin-D administration.   The patients reported that *"the discomfort in their joints had decreased"* within two weeks after beginning to take the drug.   After withdrawal of the drug, several patients complained of sharp increases in arthritic discomfort."

Note the following:

1.   Study #8 had *only 10 participants*, compared to the previous studies with up to hundreds of participants, to which *five different drugs* were given.

2.   Five of the patients were given the *impure, alcohol-extracted ergosterol* which *had already been demonstrated* in numerous studies to cause *discomfort*, which was *reversible*.   This, in effect, reduces the study down to only "five" significant patients who were taking different drugs.

3.   *The removal of calcium from their diet* at the onset of toxic symptoms (headaches and stomach aches) probably resulted in a dramatic aggravation of the symptoms as their arthritis was *caused* by calcium deficiency in the first place, and, by the authors' own admissions, "*the bones were the major source of calcium in the serum*" and not the dietary calcium.

4.   "Two" of the ten patients *(20%)* were taking calcium supplements (wafers and milk). Their symptoms were never separately identified. Were they in the "impure ergosterol" group? With so many factors, including the fact that the five individuals taking the pure vitamin-D were all on different drugs, and with so few participants, it is *impossible to draw any valid conclusions*.

5.   Although the authors reported toxic effects, the patients *all insisted* that their arthritic conditions had *dramatically improved* with the vitamin-D.

6.   In this study with so many variables on so few patients, *the results* have to be, at best, *inconclusive*, especially since they are in contradiction to the much larger studies where the variables were controlled. This study is a good example of what Dr. Reinhold Vieth calls literature about the toxicity of vitamin-D being either *"inappropriate or without substance"*.

Study #9.   --- *A Ten Year Report on the Use of Natural Food Diet With Vitamin-D* -- Roger T. Farley, M.D. and Herbert F. Spierling, M.D., *Medical Times*, **October 1948**. With the following quotes:

1)   The diet in arthritis treatment is based on the concept of fundamental physiology of nutrition: natural raw food, *unprocessed.* In all cases of arthritis, the use of white flour in any form is prohibited, and there should be no scorched fats, no creamed foods, no well cooked meals, no breaded meats, no fried foods, and no refined sugar.   Patients may have the following: all vegetables, all fruits, unroasted nuts and honey, all meats, all sea food, eggs, aged cheese, whole wheat or rye bread, and butter."

2)   In the management of arthritis, one of **the most dependable and powerful agents** on speeding the arrest and recovery **is vitamin-D**.   We began treatment (100 patients) with a   daily dosage of 50,000 I.U., increasing at 3 to 5 day periods 50,000 I.U. until indications of improvement became clear.   In the hospital, under strict management and research, we have run from 50,000 to 500,000 I.U. daily for periods of three weeks. On reduction of dosage, the *kidneys seem to have* **suffered no permanent damage,** *the urine showing no casts, no blood. In this research there has been no showing of hyper- calcemia. "*

Once again, the *effectiveness and safety* of the vitamin-D, using amounts *1,250 times* the RDA, produced by the Whittier process was proven

Study #10.   ---   *Vitamin-D: Too Much of a Good Thing* --- K.A. Fackleman, *Science News*, **May 1992.** With the following quotes:

1)   In the United States, milk has been fortified with vitamin-D since the 1930s, a policy that has greatly reduced (from 80% to practically 0%) the incidence of rickets."

2)   Ellen W. Seely and her colleagues identified 7 adults and a 15 month old girl with unexplained vitamin-D poisoning. Too much vitamin-D results in *undesirably high concentrations* of the mineral calcium in the blood which *can cause* fatigue, weight loss, and in severe cases, irreversible kidney and cardiovascular damage (no proof provided). The scientists traced the problem to milk produced by a local dairy. The Food and Drug Administration recommends that milk contain 400 I.U. of vitamin-D: however, at least one batch contained 232,565 I.U. per quart. Eleven additional cases of vitamin-D toxicity were not included in the study. However, *"the vast majority of people who drank the milk (tens of thousands) showed no sign of ill health caused by vitamin-D"*.

Note the following:

This is a typical scare tactic report which only " *suggests*" that vitamin-D "*can cause*" toxic symptoms (symptoms that are disputed as incorrect by the studies previously presented), and in this case did so (the amount consumed was *never discovered*) with 19 people, while causing *no effect* on *tens of thousands* of others. If all the people who got the high doses of vitamin-D were included in the study, the report would never have been written. Also the toxic effects induced by the vitamin-D were never described. They were probably head aches and stomach aches that stopped right after the faulty milk products were removed, or, because in proportion their numbers were so low, the milk was probably not the cause of their discomfort.

Study #11. --- *Production of 1 , 25-dihydroxy vitamin-D by Hematopoietic Cell* --- Helmut Reichel, H, Philipp Koeffler, and Anthony W. Norman, **Molecular and Cellular Regulation of Calcium and Phosphate Metabolism,** Alan R. Liss Inc, 1990, pages 81-97. With the following quotes:

1)   Vitamin-D is synthesized in the epidermis (skin) under the influence of UV light.   Alternatively, vitamin-D is provided by dietary sources. In order to become *biologically active*, vitamin-D must undergo metabolic transformation. First, vitamin-D is hydroxylated in the liver at carbon 25 to form 25-hydroxy vitamin-D, (25 (OH)D3).   The next metabolic step occurs in the   kidney   at the   1 alpha position to yield 1, 25-dihydroxytvitamin-D, 1, 25(OH)2D3, which is the biologically active vitamin-D metabolite with "*a potency that is 100 to 1000 fold higher than its precursor.*" Research by many investigators have established that 1, 25(OH)2d3 is an important hormonal regulator of calcium metabolism."

2)   The human *vitamin-D receptor, VDR*, is present in the classical *vitamin-D target intestine, bone and kidney* as well as in the parathyroid glands.   VDR is also found in the melanoma cells, breast carcinoma cells and osteosarcoma cells where 1, 25(OH)2D3 *inhibits proliferation*; in the pancreas   where 1, 25(OH)2D3 enhances the production of insulin;   in the heart muscle where 1, 25(OH)2D3

enhances ventricular contractility; and in many other organs where it plays a **crucial biological role.** "

3)   In addition to the homeostatic function of vitamin-D, there is an increasing amount of evidence that vitamin-D has important effects on tissues and organs other than those concerned with calcium homeostasis."

4)   With   regard to   the   intestinal epithelia system, the genomic effect of 1, 25(OH),D was shown several years ago when the *de vivo* synthesis of a specific vitamin-D induced   calcium-binding   protein   (calbindin-D)   was demonstrated.   In our view this appears to be an essential factor in the well documented **"enhancement of calcium absorption by vitamin-D"**

Although study #11 did not evaluate the potential toxicity of massive doses of vitamin-D, it did point out some crucial roles that vitamin-D plays in human health. Also, it introduced the **VDRs,** vitamin-D receptors, especially the VDR's in the intestines, which allow **consumed vitamin-D** with its attached mineral nutrient, to pass through the small intestine wall and therefore be absorbed by the body.

Study #12.   ---   *The Effects of Light on the Human Body* ---   Richard J. Wurtman, *Scientific American*, July 1975. With the following quotes:

The formation of vitamin-D3 or calciferol in the skin and subcutaneous tissues is the most important beneficial effect known to follow exposure to sunlight. Vitamin-D3 is formed when ultraviolet radiation is adsorbed by a precursor,

7-dehydrocholesterol. Vitamin-D2 can be found in milk and other foods and can cure rickets in children who are deficient in vitamin-D3. Investigators at the Washington University School of Medicine have concluded that *"sunlight is vastly more important than food as a source of vitamin-D3"*.

Although study #12 also did not evaluate the potential toxicity of massive doses of vitamin-D, it did point out that *sunlight* is *crucial* to the production of the more usable type of vitamin-D and therefore *sunlight is crucial to human health*. An example is *endocytosis*, which is the process that allows nutrients to be absorbed or "swallowed" by the small intestine which is covered with thousands of negatively charged, fingerlike projections called *villi*. The positive end of vitamin-D is sucked between the negative villi fingers leaving *the negative tail of the vitamin-D exposed at the surface where the positive calcium ion can attach itself*, thereby neutralizing the charge. With no negative charge left to repel the negative villi, *the villi now can wrap itself totally around the calcium-rich vitamin-D and draw the calcium deep into the base of the villi where it can be absorbed.* Once this happens, the negative end of the vitamin-D becomes exposed and is repelled to the surface by the negatively charged villi, where it is free to entrap another calcium ion and repeat the process.

And finally, a 1997 study by the North California Cancer Center concluded that *"because the skin uses ultraviolet rays from the sun to make vitamin-D* (which has been linked to protection against breast cancer in other studies which confirmed that woman from states in the tier south of Kansas tend to get significantly less breast cancer), that the *"risk of breast cancer is lowered by 40%, perhaps even more, by exposure to sunlight."*

Despite all this massive scientific evidence, the average doctor, because of drug industry propaganda *"suggesting"* vitamin-D toxicity, still believes the myth of vitamin-D toxicity. Recently, it was brought to my attention by medical pioneer, Carl Taylor, M.D., Edmonton, Canada that the medical community was constantly being bombarded with technical information *"suggesting"* that vitamin-D was toxic. Dr Taylor sent me an article entitled *"A Brief History of Vitamin-D Toxicity"*, Journal of Applied nutrition, Volume 49, Numbers 1& 2, 1997, James C. Moon, Ph.D., FACN, CNS.

Although I found the article a treasure trove of information, the article was basically *"misinformation"* as the only proof presented about the toxicity of vitamin-D was in reality *"toxicity by insinuation."* Nowhere did the article provide proof or provide statements on vitamin-D toxicity such as *"concludes that ..."* Instead, referring to vitamin-D toxicity, it used words such as *"suggests that ..."*, *"may lead to ..."* and *"may result in ..."*. These words by themselves demonstrate the lack of proof in this article of the toxicity of vitamin-D. By using the phrase *"excessive vitamin-D may lead to hypercalcemia"*, vitamin -D is then held responsible for the damage to health caused by hypercalcemia, when in fact, just the opposite is true. High serum calcium levels are a direct result of decalcification of the bones for the purpose of supplying calcium to the organs which are desperate for calcium. *It is also due to a lack of sunshine, resulting in low calcium regulating calcitonin production and calcium storage inisotol triphosphate production.* Calcium deficiencies, due to lack of calcium in the diet along with lack of vitamin-D, are *"responsible for hypercalcemia"*.

 Vitamin-D, produced by sunshine, allows the body to absorb large quantities of calcium and therefore helps to prevent hypercalcemia. Furthermore, the sunshine that produces the vitamin-D also causes the pituitary gland to instruct the parathyroid gland to produce the hormone calcitonin, which prevents the decalcification of the bones. Thus, vitamin-D *actually prevents the very health problems that it is accused of causing*. The scientific studies that *"suggested"* otherwise did not include the other numerous health factors that play a major role in hypercalcemia. None of these studies meet the basic requirement of being *"multi year, phase 1, 2 and 3, double blind and massive studies done on large numbers of individuals"*, that are requirements to scientifically determine toxicity. The article would therefore not withstand scrutiny from scientific peers and was probably paid for by the drug industry.

 Typical of articles attempting to perpetuate the myth that God's nutrient, vitamin-D, is toxic, the article not only provides misinformation, it also uses arguments that are not true. For example, it states that "there have been no systematic studies to determine vitamin-D toxicity for humans". In the previous pages I have provided 12 such studies, *"all"* of which *"conclude that vitamin-D is not toxic."* Many of these were ten year studies done on hundreds of animals and humans. Studies that were carried out by our best scientists and doctors at our best scientific research establishments. For example, the Streck Report of 1937, *"Further Studies on Intoxification With Vitamin-D"*, which was done at the University of Chicago Medical Facility and took dozens of doctors and scientists nine years to complete, concluded that they found large doses of vitamin-D to be non toxic and, because of the correlation of their animal studies to their human studies, they concluded that *"the burden of proof rests with those who claim the undesirability of vitamin-D therapy"*. This study was followed up by other massive studies which all concluded the "non toxicity of vitamin-D". Therefore, the claim of no systematic studies to determine vitamin-D toxicity *is fraudulent* and results in great harm to the health of America.

Finally, this article did provide information that proved that vitamin-D, in the amounts such as 1200 IU and 2000 IU which they claimed were toxic, just simply could not possibly be toxic. It is simple because all one has to do is apply grade 8 math to the numbers provided in the article. The article refers to a paper *"Cholecalciferol Production"*, P.C. Beadle, where Beadle measured the vitamin-D production in the epidermis (skin) to be *163 IU per square centimeter* in *light skin* per day and *69 IU per square centimeter in dark skin* per day.

The human body has about 20 square feet of skin or 18,600 square centimeters. This means that the human body can produce over *3,000,000 IU of non toxic vitamin-D per day*. Therefore, if the article had any merit, we all would be dead after exposure to more than one minute of sunlight, and yet they suggest we all get at least 30 minutes per week.

Also, the article suggests that 30 minutes of sunshine per week produces enough vitamin-D for the human body. Assuming this to be true, and also assuming the sun shines for at least 12 hours per day, the amount of vitamin-D produced in 30 minutes is 128,000 IU which when taken over a 7 day week, calculates to "18,300 IU per day". This means that they are advising that "18,300 IU of vitamin-D is required by the human body per day" (which this author wholeheartedly supports), while saying, at the same time, that 1200 IU "may be toxic". Apparently the author of the article has trouble with grade school math. *Which is it, 18,000 or 1,200?* The latter is ludicrous as the healthiest people in the world, *the Hunzas in Pakistan, the Bamas in China, the Georgians in Russia, the Titi Cacas in Peru and the Okinawans in Japan*, all of whom have virtually no diseases, all get about 7 hours of sunshine each day and therefore produce about 500,000 IU of Vitamin-D each day (their skin is dark). Thus, the logic of the Ph.D.'s who apparently cannot calculate, lies in the ruins of grade eight math.

Therefore, the publication, *A brief History of Vitamin-D Toxicity* is another example of Dr. Veith's literature citations being either inappropriate or without substance. This article definitely is based on both.

Other interesting studies have been done. *The Lancet*, Garland et al, February 9, 1985 issue reported that a long study had shown that men with the *highest vitamin-D in the blood had 1.42% colon cancer whereas those with the lowest had 3.89 % (or 273% more cancer).* *The Lancet*, Garland et al, November 18, 1989 issue reported a study of 25,000 in Maryland showed that there was *80% more colon cancers in the fifth of the population with the lowest vitamin-D in the blood.* In a report from England, *The Lancet,* March 23, 1991 stated that 3 of 14 women who were treated with *topical vitamin-D experienced a reduction of 50% in their malignant breast tumors.* A report in *Cancer*, 70, 1992, pp2861-9, by C.C. Hanchette and G.G. Schartz entitled *"Geographic Patterns of Prostate Cancer mortality, Evidence for Protective Effect of Ultraviolet Radiation"* notes that areas in **Northern latitudes, such as Iceland, Denmark and Sweden have far more prostate cancers than found in areas of more intense sunlight.** A report from M. Frydenburg of the Urology Department in the Royal Melbourne Hospital in *Cancer Forum,* Vol.19, No 1, March 1995, pp 15-18, states that **high vitamin-D in the blood may be protective for prostate cancer.**

In conclusion, medical doctors are reading and believing the thesis that vitamin-D is toxic, and as a result, are **"perpetuating disease".** Ironically, I know medical doctors who claim to have treated patients suffering from vitamin-D toxicity. This only proves to demonstrate the medical fact that **"at least 50% of all medical diagnoses are incorrect".** Therefore, the use of vitamin-D with calcium supplementation could make a major impact on the war against disease.

CHAPTER 10

The Newspaper History & the Suppression of Vitamins

When a story becomes controversial such as the 95 year story of vitamins, in order to understand what is the truth, one has to research for appropriate documents. One of the best sources of the truth is the newspapers of the time which report third party opinion. When you read these stories you will see that today, all of the government regulatory agencies, which are puppets of the drug industry, are taking the stance that no one should be allowed to make medical claims on vitamins. They want us to believe that vitamins are drugs that should be regulated by the FDA (drug industry puppet), and that vitamins should only be sold by prescriptions regulated by the AMA (drug industry puppet).

You will see as you read the newspaper stories that these agencies have taken this position for the past 95 years, and refuse to change. On the other hand, thousands of medical researchers along with the nutrition industry have concluded that vitamins both prolong life and inhibit a host of diseases, including cancer, diabetes and MS. This is very ironic, because all government agencies are perpetually trying to suppress vitamins. *If the drug industry had just one drug that worked as well as any vitamin, that drug would be worth trillions of dollars today.* No such drug exists, as the drug industry has failed to compete with God's nutrients. Despite this, the newspapers tell a story of government agencies perpetually attempting to discredit vitamins and to put them under the control of the drug industry. These agencies have lost in the courts and also lost in Congress, but they refuse to give up and continue to waste the taxpayers' money. Obviously, the heads of these agencies should be replaced by people who know how to use logic and who would represent the best interests of the people.

For example, the FDA should do its duty and not just evaluate drugs but also evaluate food by examining the massive scientific documentation on how vitamins and minerals enhance human health, and then perform their duty by issuing hundreds of FDA approved scientific claims for God's Nutrients. Millions have died and millions more will die because this is not happening.

Jun 20, 1922
FIND SUN PRODUCES THE 4TH VITAMIN; Columbia Professors Discover Rickets May Be Cured Without Use of Cod Liver Oil.
NO CHANGE OF DIET NEEDED Analysis of Patients Show

Mysterious Effect of Sunlight Upon the Blood.
New York Times (1857-Current file). New York, N.Y.: June 20, 1922. pg. 18, 1 pgs

Abstract (Document Summary)

While the study of rickets at *Johns Hopkins University has resulted in the discovery reported yesterday of a fourth type of vitamin (Vitamin D),* the study of rickets at the *College of Physicians and Surgeons of Columbia University has indicated that sunlight may produce vitamins directly in the human blood.*

Comment: **This was the first time that it was recognized that sunshine can produce a vitamin.**

Jun 22, 1922

DR. FUNK IN SEARCH OF SIXTH VITAMIN; Discoverer of the One Necessary to Life Predicts More Will Be Found.
EXPLAINS RESEARCH WORK
Fifth Chemical Factor Found at Johns Hopkins--List Now Runs From A to E. Process of Separation. Studied by Belgians. The List of Vitamins.
New York Times (1857-Current file). New York, N.Y.: Jun 22, 1922. pg. 7, 1 pgs

Abstract (Document Summary)

Dr. Casimir Funk, who ten years ago discovered the mysterious unidentified chemical factors necessary to life for which he invented the name of vitamins, explained yesterday his discovery of Vitamin D. Dr. Funk is the head of the laboratories of ex-Controller Herman A. Metz, ...

Comment: **Dr. Funk was responsible for the name "vitamins".**

Mar 23, 1924
VITAMIN DISCOVERY STIRS SCIENTISTS; Isolation of "D" Opens Up Possibility of Producing Nutritive Synthetic Food.

New York Times (1857-Current file). New York, N.Y.: Mar 23, 1924. pg. E5, 1 pgs

Abstract (Document Summary)

Unusual interest has been aroused in medical circles by the announcement of *Dr. Walter H. Eddy. Professor of Physiological Chemistry in Teachers College, Columbia University, of the first isolation of any of the five known vitamins.* Dr. Eddy and his associates believe that isolation of Vitamin D or, as Dr. Eddy prefers, "Blos" opens up the possibility of producing synthetic foods of a high nutritive value...

Comment: This was the first time that vitamin-D was isolated.

Feb 19, 1928
'SUNSHINE' SOLD IN PILLS IN BRITAIN; Vitamin D. Produced by Action of Ultra-Violet Light, Is Achieved by Synthesis.

Special Correspondence of THE NEW YORK TIMES.. **New York Times (1857-Current file)**. New York, N.Y.: Feb 19, 1928. pg. 56, 1 pgs

Abstract (Document Summary)

LONDON, Feb. 11--*"Sunshine" can now be taken medicinally in a pill.* Vitamin D, which has been described as the *"sunshine vitamin" because it comes from the sun, can now be bought in small pellets.*

Comment: This was the turning point in the history of drugs versus vitamins, because, for the first time, the public could consume large quantities of vitamin-D. The result became a medical emergency as people began curing disease and the hospitals began to empty. The men of medicine had to do something to end this trend, so they decided to give seven medical students enough vitamin-D to kill a horse. It worked as the students got sick and the medical authorities immediately had vitamin-D removed from the selves of America. As there were other vitamins, such as vitamin-A and vitamin-E that apparently had merit in preventing disease, the men of medicine decided that they would institute a program of propaganda against these vitamins. They decided on a program of numbers psychology. They would change the units of measurement of vitamins A, D and E from milligrams to a new unit called "International Units" or IUs. It worked as the small amount of 20 milligrams of vitamin-D became 1,000,000 IUs, an amount that the public deemed to be horrifically high as when they ate an orange they only got 60 milligrams of vitamin-C. The medical recommendation of 400 IUs seemed high enough, even though it was only 1/100th of a milligram, an amount to small to be effective. Thus the public to this day are being duped by psychology into thinking that they are getting adequate amounts of vitamins, when in reality, the amounts recommended by the medical authorities are criminally low.

Back in 1928, there was a public outcry about the removal of vitamin-D due to its toxicity. As a result, the University of Chicago Medical Faculty was commissioned to study vitamin-D toxicity. It took dozens of doctors and scientists ten years to conclude in their final report, the Frock Report, that no amount of vitamin-D was toxic and that the medical claims pf cures were true. The public, by this time, had almost forgotten about vitamin-D but the drug industry saw profits so they created four of the most popular drugs of all times that were merely vitamin-D placebos, such as Dalsol, Deltalin, Drisdol. The result, other that staggering profits, was that the public began to believe that some drugs actually work. In the meantime the men of medicine still warned the public that anything more than 400IU daily "could be toxic" even though they prescribed Drugs in the hundreds of thousands of IUs of vitamin-D his practice continues to this day.

April 3, 1929

TELLS OF NEW DRUG AS RICKETS CURE; Dr. A.F. Hess *Says Irradiated Ergosterol Acts Like Taking Ultra-Violet Rays.* **THERAPEUTIC USE DELAYED** Dosage Has Not Yet Been Fully Established, American Institute Is Informed.

New York Times (1857-Current file). New York, N.Y.: Apr

3, 1929. pg. 37, 1 pgs

Abstract (Document Summary)

Science has in its possession a new drug which is *"many thousand times as potent as the well known cod liver oil"* and which *when exposed to ultra-violet rays creates Vitamin D and is empowered with a remarkable* ...

Comment: In other words, vitamin-D cures the horrific childhood disease, Rickets.

May 31, 1929

SAYS SUN'S RAYS AID HEALTH ENTIRE YEAR; Dr. Riddle Tells Tuberculosis Association Idea of Benefit in Summer Only Is Wrong.

Special to The New York Times.. **New York Times (1857-Current file)**. New York, N.Y.: May 31, 1929. pg. 44, 1 pgs

Abstract (Document Summary)

ATLANTIC CITY, N.J., May 30.-- *Healthful qualities of sunshine are found in the rays at all times of the sun* ...

Comment: In other words, the vitamin-D produced by the sun all year round helped those with one of the most dreaded diseases of the time, tuberculosis.

Jan 15, 1931

CREATES VITAMIN D BY SELECTIVE RAYS; Dr. Sperti of Cincinnati Finds Only Small Part of Ultra- Violet Band Effective. *Milk Can Now Be Treated Without Spoiling,* He Says--Discovery, Called Important. Dr. Sperti Explains Researches. Effect of Different Rays.

New York Times (1857-Current file). New York, N.Y.: Jan 15, 1931. pg. 22, 1 pgs

Abstract (Document Summary)

Discovery of how to irradiate Vitamin D by the application of selective ultra-violet rays, regarded by experts as likely to have an important bearing on the increase of the nutritive and health-building properties...

Comment: In other words, the medical researchers of 1931 believed that Vitamin-D was so nutritional to the benefit of health that they recommended that it be put in foods such as milk.

Feb 12, 1931
PRODUCE NEW BREAD WITH VITAMIN "D"; Toronto Doctors Find Source of Health-Giving Element to Supplement Sunshine.

Special to The New York Times.. **New York Times (1857-Current file)**. New York, N.Y.: Feb 12, 1931. pg. 2, 1 pgs

Abstract (Document Summary)

TORONTO, Feb. 11.--*Conclusions that vitamin D is essential to normal human metabolism; that a large percentage of people in the, temperate zone obtain very little vitamin D through its chief source, sunshine, and that an additional general supply of the vitamin may be made.*

Comment: Thus vitamin-D was added to one of the most popular foods, bread.

Feb 13, 1931
MILLION REPORTED BID FOR VITAMIN D RIGHTS; Toronto Authorities Decline to Confirm Story of Offer by American 'Interests.'

Special to The New York Times.. **New York Times (1857-Current file)**. New York, N.Y.: Feb 13, 1931. pg. 21, 1 pgs

Abstract (Document Summary)

TORONTO, Feb. 12.--Reports were current here today that *$1,000,000 had been offered for the right to use the process by which ordinary bread is charged with "Sunshine Vitamin D."* The offer, it was said, was made by interests in the United States to authorities at the University of Toronto, which controls the process.

Comment: To put things in perspective $1,000,000 in 1931 is equivalent to over $30,000,000 in 2005 dollars. That means that in 1931, big time money was spent on the rights to use vitamin-D in bread, so this means that there must have been a consensus that vitamin-D worked so well at improving human health that huge sums of money should be spent on the acquisition to rights to use the vitamin.

Mar 10, 1931

VITAMIN D RIGHTS BOUGHT FOR BREAD; Chain Bakers Here to Use **'Sunshine' Product**, Prepared in the Laboratory of Toronto University.

Special to The New York Times.. **New York Times (1857-Current file)**. New York, N.Y.: Mar 10, 1931. pg. 20, 1 pgs

Comment: This means that the bread industry in the US believed in the health benefits of vitamin-D

May 8, 1931CONFERENCE ON VITAMINS HERE; 26 Experts Meet to Set Standards for Medicinal Products.

New York Times (1857-Current file). New York, N.Y.: May 8, 1931. pg. 2, 1 pgs

Comment: In other words, consideration for vitamins had become a big time.

Jul 5, 1931
VITAMINS PLAY A BIG ROLE IN SUSTAINING OUR HEALTH; The Six Now Known Are Interdependent in the Benefits They Bestow Upon Mankind--that What We Know of Them *Vitamin A. Vitamin B. Vitamin C. Vitamin D. Vitamin E.*

By H.C. SHERMAN, Mitchill Professor of Chemistry, Columbia University.. **New York Times (1857-Current file)**. New York, N.Y.: Jul 5, 1931. pg. 96, 2 pgs

Abstract (Document Summary)

RESEARCH has established the fact that normal nutrition requires a group of substances different from the long-familiar proteins, fats, carbohydrates and mineral matters. *These recently apprehended substances are at present collectively called "vitamins"*

Comment: It therefore appears that the support for the "big role of vitamins in sustaining good health that was being exposed by medical researchers, was being recognized and supported by the press in 1931.

Nov 21, 1931
German Nobel Prize Chemist Makes Crystals of Vitamin D

New York Times (1857-Current file). New York, N.Y.: Nov 21, 1931. pg. 1, 1 pgs

Nov 24, 1931
POISON IN BIG DOSE OF PURE VITAMIN D; German Makes Discovery in His Work of Four Years Producing Isolation.
FIND CLEARS A MOOT POINT Professor Adolf Windaus

Proves Ill Effects Do Not Come From a Mingled Substance.

New York Times (1857-Current file). New York, N.Y.: Nov 24, 1931. pg. 27, 1 pgs

Abstract (Document Summary)

BERLIN, Nov. 23 (AP).--*Pure Vitamin D is a poison as well as a lifesaver*. This discovery was explained today as one result of the *"isolation" of a crystal which is pure Vitamin D,* announced last week by Professor Adolf Windaus.

Comment: In other words, vitamin-D research was so important in 1931 that Nobel Prize winners were participating.

Dec 31, 1931
SYNTHETIC VITAMINS.

New York Times (1857-Current file). New York, N.Y.: Dec 31, 1931. pg. 11, 1 pgs

Abstract (Document Summary)

Only a few weeks ago Vitamin D, which prevents rickets, was isolated in the laboratories of WINDAUS in Germany, REERINK and VAN WIJK in ...

Comment: Thus scientists in Germany were working on vitamin-D in 1931

Jan 4, 1932
Scientists in London Claim Isolation of Pure Vitamin D

By The Associated Press.. **New York Times (1857-Current file)**. New York, N.Y.: Jan 4, 1932. pg. 14, 1 pgs

Comment: Thus scientists in England were also working on vitamin-D. in 1932.

May 22, 1932
NEW FINDINGS ABOUT VITAMINS STRESS THE EFFECT OF LIGHT; Synthetic Production of Life-Fostering Substances Brought Nearer as a Result of Ultraviolet Ray Experiments

By WALDEMAR KAEMPFFERT.. **New York Times (1857-Current file)**. New York, N.Y.: May 22, 1932. pg. XX4, 1 pgs

Abstract (Document Summary)

ALTHOUGH vitamins are not the discovery of any one man, there can be no doubt that it was *Sir Frederick Gowland Hopkins of Cambridge, England, president of the Royal Society and Nobel prize winner, who drove home to physicians the importance of the few that were known twenty year ago and stimulated research in a branch of chemistry which is revealing more and more* ...

Comment: Dr. Robert R. Williams in 1910 along with Dr. Casmir Funk in 1912 were the first to recognize the existence of vitamins. It was considered so important that he was joined in his research efforts by Nobel Prize winner Sir Frederick Gowland Hopkins, President of the Royal Society. Both men agreed how essential sun on the skin was to the production of the crucial vitamin-D.

Jun 24, 1932
LONGER LIFE BASED ON DIET ELEMENTS; *Calcium and Phosphorus In the Right Ratio Can Make Span 77 Years,* Scientists Are Told. **OLD AGE HASTENED BY LACK**

From a Staff Correspondent Special to THE NEW YORK TIMES.. **New York Times (1857-Current file)**. New York, N.Y.: Jun 24, 1932. pg. 10, 1 pgs

Abstract (Document Summary)

SYRACUSE, N. Y., June 23.-- Evidence that old age could be greatly postponed and that the *span of human life might be increased from the traditional three score and ten (70 years) to three score and seventeen (78 years) by the intake of the proper proportions of calcium and phosphorus in the diet* was presented here today before the Summer meeting of the American Association for the Advancement of ...

Comment: It therefore appears that in 1932 scientist had determined that the mineral calcium can extend life. Of course this cannot occur without the assistance of calcium's biological partner, vitamin-D. The drug industry of the time must have been reeling from the revelation that a food substance, calcium, and not a drug was the answer to longevity.

Jul 29, 1932

VITAMIN D ISOLATED IN NATURAL FORM; *Tasteless Product Is Extracted From Cod Liver Oil* by Prof. T.F. Zucker of Columbia. **IT CAN BE USED IN FOODS** Process Patented by University to Prevent Exploitation -- *Value In Curing Rickets Described.*

New York Times (1857-Current file). New York, N.Y.: Jul 29, 1932. pg. 17, 1 pgs

Abstract (Document Summary)

A process for the *extraction of pure Vitamin D directly from cod liver oil has been perfected at Columbia University by Professor Theodore F. Zucker after ten years of research and experimentation,* it was announced yesterday at the university.

Comment: What is important is that the scientific community recognized the importance of vitamin-D to health and were working to prevent its exploitation. This process to produce vitamin-D was less expensive than others and therefore provided hope for an inexpensive supply.

Dec 7, 1932

PROVE VITAMIN D HALTS TOOTH DECAY; Dr. and Mrs. Agnew, Honored at Luncheon, Tell of Research With Rats and Children. **PHOSPHOROUS ALSO VITAL** Experiments at Toronto Indicate Sweets Affect Teeth Only by Restricting Normal Diet.

New York Times (1857-Current file). New York, N.Y.: Dec 7, 1932. pg. 24, 1 pgs

Abstract (Document Summary)

Tooth decay, the common malady of civilized man, is primarily due to a lack of phosphorus in the diet and *a lack of vitamin D, obtained when the skin is exposed to sunshine or by the consumption of fish oils*, it was shown definitely through researches carried on by Dr. R. Gordon Agnew of the faculty of West China Union University and revealed by him ...

Comment: Since calcium, which is crucial to the health of the tooth, is the biological partner to vitamin-D, these scientific findings that vitamin-D prevents cavities should not come as surprise.

Mar 11, 1934

OSTEOPATHS TOLD OF VITAMIN VALUE; Dr. S.L. Davis Says *Lack of Them in Food Coincides With High Death Rate Curve.* **DESIRABLE DIET GIVEN** Posture Emphasized by Dr. E.R. Hoskins at Convention of Eastern Group Here.

New York Times (1857-Current file). New York, N.Y.: Mar 11, 1934. pg. N1, 1 pgs

Abstract (Document Summary)

Vitamins partaken of in adequate quantities "prolong the span of life", while the lack of them in the human body, particularly of vitamins A and D, are responsible for many Winter ills and often directly cause an early death, Dr. S.L. Davis, director of the Washington Research Foundation, told the annual convention of the

Eastern Osteopathic Association yesterday.

Comment: Thus, the scientific community in 1934 concluded that vitamins prolong human life.

Dec 9, 1935

BIG VITAMIN D DOSES GIVEN FOR ARTHRITIS; Successful Treatment of the Disease Is Reported by Two Illinois University Doctors.

New York Times (1857-Current file). New York, N.Y.: Dec 9, 1935. pg. 23, 1 pgs

Abstract (Document Summary)

CHICAGO, Dec. 8 (AP). – "*Successful treatment for arthritis with great doses of Vitamin D*" was described today by Dr. C.I. Reed, of the University of Illinois College of Medicine.

Comment: Therefore, as other scientists of the time had discovered, these two University of Illinois doctors concluded that vitamin-D, "in great doses" could be used successfully to treat arthritis. Dr. Frock, University of Chicago Medical Faculty also made the same conclusion in his 1938 report. Therefore scientists of the day were continuing to conclude that vitamin-D cures disease.

Mar 26, 1936

POTENT VITAMIN D FOUND IN FISH OILS; Illinois Study Yields Type Much More Powerful in Fighting Poultry Rickets. **G' MAY BAR CATARACTS '** Significant' Relation to Their Growth Seen in Report to Nutritionists at Capital.

By WILLIAM L. LAUBENCE Special to THE NEW YORK TIMES.. **New York Times (1857-Current file).** New York, N.Y.: Mar 26, 1936. pg. 7, 1 pgs

Abstract (Document Summary)

122

WASHINGTON, March 25. -- *Discovery of a new type of vitamin D in fish oils,* and synthesis of the new vitamin in the laboratory, were announced today before the American Institute of Nutrition. .

Comment: **Thus other scientists continue to extol the health virtues of vitamin-D**

Apr 6, 1936
FIND VITAMIN D AIDS DIGESTIVE PROCESS; M.I.T. *Experimenters Learn That It Tends to Offset Intestinal Sluggishness.*
New York Times (1857-Current file). New York, N.Y.: Apr 6, 1936. pg. 22, 1 pgs

Abstract (Document Summary)

CAMBRIDGE, Mass., April 5 (AP). -- *Experiments which suggest an unexpected value to humans in vitamin D* were made public today at the Massachusetts Institute of Technology.

Comment: **The scientists in 1936, although recognizing the importance of vitamin-D to the digestive system, did not know about the vitamin-D receptors or VDRs that lined the intestine resulting in a dramatic absorption of nutrients.**

Aug 23, 1936
THE WEEK IN SCIENCE: A SYNTHETIC 'NERVE VITAMIN'; Scientists Produce Basic Food Factor B1 Artificially -- New Step in Hormones
By WILLIAM L. LAURENCE. **New York Times (1857-Current file).** New York, N.Y.: Aug 23, 1936. pg. XX4, 1 pgs

Abstract (Document Summary)

TWENTY-SIX years ago Dr. Robert R. Williams, who since has become chemical director of the Bell Telephone Laboratories, began to devote his spare time to the *study and investigation of vitamin B1*, generally known as the *"nerve vitamin" because of its importance in keeping nerve tissue in a healthy state.*

Comment: It therefore appears that another crucial vitamin, B1, can be added to the list of vitamins that result in dramatic improvements to human health. This meant that the medical authorities of the day had to keep this crucial information from their drug dispensing doctors.

Sep 9, 1936
VITAMIN A IS FOUND TO ATTACK DISEASE; Mobilized From the Liver to Points Where Most Needed, Chemists Are Told. **ORANGE REAMING IS URGED** Californian Declares That This Gives More Vitamin C Than Squeezing Method.

Special to THE NEW YORK TIMES.. **New York Times (1857-Current File).** New York, N.Y.: Sep 9, 1936. pg. 23, 1 pgs

Abstract (Document Summary)

PITTSBURGH, Sept. 8. -- Discussion *concerning the vitamins necessary to physical wellbeing had a large share in the doings of the American Chemical Society today* **Comment:** Thus, the prestigious Chemical Society of 1936 joins the chorus of medical researchers claiming that vitamins both attack and cure disease. Four decades later a Nobel prize was issued to Linus Pauling who better elucidated the claim.

Apr 15, 1937
PUREST VITAMIN A MADE BY CHEMIST; Crystal Form of

Life-Giving Substance Is Shown by Holmes of Oberlin

By *WILLIAM L. LAURENCE, Special to THE NEW YORK TIMES.*. **New York Times (1857-Current file)**. New York, N.Y.: Apr 15, 1937. pg. 26, 1 pgs

Abstract (Document Summary)

Isolation at last of vitamin A in pure crystalline form, with an increase in potency of 1,000,000 vitamin units above the best present concentrates, was announced today before the meeting of the American Chemical Society at the University of North Carolina.

Comment: **It therefore appears that the best scientists of 1937 were giving best efforts to the production of purer vitamins.**

Apr 27, 1939

WASTE IS DEPLORED IN VITAMIN FOODS; Nutritionists at Toronto Are Told Low Income Families Cannot Get All Benefits $100,000,000 A YEAR SPENT Too Great an Addition Also Is Pictured as Possibly Harmful 'Shotgun' Prophylaxis

By *WILLIAM L. LAURENCE Special to THE NEW YORK TIMES.*. **New York Times (1857-Current File)**. New York, N.Y.: Apr 27, 1939. pg. 37, 1 pgs

Abstract (Document Summary)

TORONTO, Ont., April 26.*-- American people spent last year a sum estimated at more than $100,000,000 for vitamin preparations,* in the belief that their health would thereby be greatly improved and dire ills be prevented.

Comment: **It should be noted that $100,000,000 in 1939 is equivalent to $1,100,000,000 in 2005 dollars. Hence that drug industry was eager to share in this money and so, after it learned from the Frock report that vitamin-D did indeed prevent disease, it began the production of its own best selling vitamin-D drugs, Dalsol, Deltalin, Drisdol.**

May 20, 1939

VITAMIN K IS USED FOR COAGULATION; *Prevention of Hemorrhages in Surgery* on Jaundiced Patients Is Reported to Doctors **OPERATIVE RISK REDUCED** *Substance, Normal in Body, Found in Plants, Starts Chain Forming Thrombin in Blood*

By WILLIAM L. LAURENCE Special to THE NEW YORK TIMES.. **New York Times (1857-Current file).** New York, N.Y.: May 20, 1939. pg. 12, 1 pgs

Abstract (Document Summary)

ST. LOUIS, May 19.--*The saving of the lives of many jaundiced patients in need of surgical operations by the administration of the still mysterious coagulation vitamin*, which has so far eluded all ...

Comment: Thus another use was found for another vitamin.

Mar 31, 1941

VITAMINS AND WAR

New York Times (1857-Current file). New York, N.Y.: Mar 31, 1941. pg. 14, 1 pgs

Abstract (Document Summary)

Even physicians are hardly aware of the "revolution in nutrition" which was brought about by the last war and which is still in progress. Very little was known about vitamins in 1915. Indeed, the word had not even passed into medical vernacular. Nevertheless, *British experts were already beginning to think of vitamins in terms of deficiency diseases,* whereas the Germans could see nothing in food ...

Comment: Thus, wartime Europe recognized the significance of vitamins to human health, referring to the "revolution in nutrition".

Jun 16, 1941
EXPERTS TO STUDY NEW VITAMIN IDEAS; They Will Discuss Value of Enriching Foods as Has Been Done With Bread
LOSSES BY COOKING CITED: Dr. S.C. Prescott Says Home-Makers Must Be Trained to Preserve Natural Content

By MARGOT MURPHY Special to THE NEW YORK TIMES.. **New York Times (1857-Current file)**. New York, N.Y.: Jun 16, 1941. pg. 10, 1 pgs

Abstract (Document Summary)

PITTSBURGH, June 15 -- *Possible fortification of additional everyday foods with vitamins is a subject uppermost in the minds of members of the Institute of Food Technologists,* gathering here for their second annual conference, which is scheduled to open tomorrow morning.

Comment: **It therefore appears that the medical authorities became mortal enemies of the Institute of Food Technologists who were attempting to put more vitamins in more food.**

Sep 15, 1941
VITAMIN C LINKED TO REPRODUCTION; Wisconsin Biochemists Report to Symposium That It Acts to Postpone Senescence
EFFECTIVE UPON CATTLE; Preliminary Tests on Human Beings Show Results Except in Pathological Sterility

By WILLIAM L. LAURENCE special to THE NEW YORK TIMES.. **New York Times (1857-Current file)**. New York, N.Y.: Sep 15, 1941. pg. 19, 1 pgs

Abstract (Document Summary)

MADISON, Wis., Sept. 14 -- The discovery *that Vitamin C, essential for the prevention of scurvy and for the maintenance of healthy gums, teeth and capillaries, also plays a vital role in reproduction was announced today at the University of Wisconsin,* following a three-day symposium on the respiratory enzymes.

Comment: Another gold star for another vitamin, vitamin-A proving to be important in reproduction.

May 3, 1942

What We Know About Vitamins; *As new vitamins are found so are new deficiencies in food, and nutrition becomes part of preventive medicine.*

By WALDEMAR KAEMPFFERT. **New York Times (1857-Current file)**. New York, N.Y.: May 3, 1942. pg. SM10, 3 pgs

Abstract (Document Summary)

EVEN before we decided to arm ourselves to the teeth, we knew that all was not well with the American diet. *A mild popular interest in vitamins which began twenty years ago has developed into a wave of nutritional reform. The health of the nation of the armed forces, of the workers in munitions plants depends on them.*

Comment: War time America began recognizing the importance of vitamins to human health.

Apr 14, 1943

VITAMIN A APPLIED TO WHOOPING COUGH; Chemists Are Told of Tests Showing Rat Recovery -- Body Found to Store Factor

By WILLIAM L. LAURENCE Special to THE NEW YORK TIMES.. **New York Times (1857-Current file)**. New York, N.Y.: Apr 14, 1943. pg. 46, 1 pgs

Abstract (Document Summary)

DETROIT, April 13 -- Experiments showing *that vitamin A saves the lives of animals infected with whooping cough, one of the most serious diseases of children, and the further discovery that a protein constituent enables the body to store a supply of this essential vitamin for emergency uses,* were reported today before the meeting of the American Chemical Society.

Comment: Another use for another vitamin is recognized by the prestigious American Chemical Society, much to the distress of the drug industry.

Jul 2, 1943

VITAMIN D PATENTS VOIDED; Federal Appeals Court Finds Nature Source of Wisconsin Process Yielding $7,500,000

By LAWRENCE E. DAVIES, Special to THE NEW YORK TIMES.. **New York Times (1857-Current file).** New York, N.Y.: Jul 2, 1943. pg. 17, 1 pgs

Abstract (Document Summary)

SAN FRANCISCO, July 1 -- *Patents covering production of vitamin D, reported to have yielded royalties exceeding $7,500,000 to the University of Wisconsin Alumni Research Foundation,* were held invalid today by the Federal Circuit Court of Appeals.

Comment: Once again it is interesting to not that the $7,500,000 in 1943 dollars is equivalent to $83,000,000 in 2005 dollars which is a handsome sum for a royalty for anything. Once again in 1943, vitamin-D was a top news story.

Jul 18, 1943

MOVE FOR REVERSAL IN VITAMIN D SUIT; Wisconsin Alumni Foundation Trustees Decide to Contest Invalidating of Patent

Special to THE NEW YORK TIMES.. **New York Times (1857-Current file).** New York, N.Y.: Jul 18,

1943. pg. 36, 1 pgs

Abstract (Document Summary)

CHICAGO, July 17 -- Trustees of the *Wisconsin Alumni Research Foundation* decided today to ask the Ninth Circuit Court of Appeals at San Francisco to *restudy a ruling declaring that valuable patents covering the manufacture of Vitamin D are invalid.*

Comment: Once again the importance of vitamin-D patents is covered by the American press.

Oct 22, 1943

CHARGES VITAMIN D IS IN TIGHT CONTROL; Berge of Justice Department Tells Senators a Research Group Is Monopoly Screen

Special to THE NEW YORK TIMES.. **New York Times (1857-Current   file).** New   York,   N.Y.: Oct   22, 1943. pg. 13, 1 pgs

Abstract (Document Summary)

WASHINGTON, Oct. 21 -- A charge that the *Wisconsin Alumni Research Foundation instead of keeping to its announced purpose of protecting the public against "unscrupulous commercialism" had been led by love of profit to act "as a screen behind which a group of monopolistic chemical, pharmaceutical and food companies control vitamin D"* was made before the Senate War Mobilization subcommittee today by Wendell Berge, Assistant ...

Comment: Once again, the importance of vitamin-D had been brought up in congress   as it had been recognized that the chemical, pharmaceutical and food companies   had   all   been making huge profits on the sale of vitamin-D.

May 7, 1944

A Cure for Deficiency Diseases

W.K.. **New York Times (1857-Current file)**. New York, N.Y.: May 7, 1944. pg. E9, 1 pgs

Abstract (Document Summary)

At last week's exercises in commemoration of the *125th anniversary of the University of Cincinnati the principal address was delivered by Dr. Tom D. Spies, noted for his clinical researches in pellagra and other diseases caused by a deficiency of some vitamin.* He gave his hearers not only a summary of what bad eating habits can do to any man or woman but also the ...

Comment: **It therefore appears that the medical experts of 1944 recognized that many diseases were caused by vitamin deficiencies.**

Jun 24, 1944

Vitamin Tablets Are Ruled Drugs And General Sale in State Curbed; STATE CURBS SALE OF VITAMIN PILLS

Special to THE NEW YORK TIMES.. **New York Times (1857-Current file)**. New York, N.Y.: Jun 24, 1944. pg. 1, 2 pgs

Abstract (Document Summary)

ALBANY, June 23 -- **Attorney General Nathaniel L. Goldstein ruled today that vitamins,** when listed in the official United States Pharmacopoeia or national formulary, *were drugs and could be sold at retail only by registered pharmacists, drug stores and registered stores.*

Comment: **Therefore, for the first time, the medical authorities, had found a way to eliminate competition in the sale of vitamins, by simply having vitamins declared a drug. This would also give more control to restricting the amounts of vitamins and thereby ensuring the proliferation both of disease and their drug profits.**

Jun 25, 1944

VITAMIN SALES BAN MAY LAND IN COURT; Grocers Studying Decision of Attorney General, Hint at Possible Legal Test

New York Times (1857-Current file). New York, N.Y.: Jun 25, 1944. pg. 32, 1 pgs

Abstract (Document Summary)

A court test of State *Attorney General Nathaniel L. Goldstein's ruling that concentrated vitamins may be sold only by pharmacists or in stores* registered by the State Board of Pharmacy appeared likely yesterday as *grocers protested that the ruling would give drug stores a virtual monopoly in this State on a business that amounts throughout the nation to $250,000,000 a year*

Comment: One should note that $250.000,000 in 1944 is equal to $5,817,000,000 in 2005 dollars, giving the drug industry financial cause to suppress vitamins that were definitely competing with their drug sales.

Oct 21, 1944

17 MORE FIRMS PUT IN VITAMIN D SUIT; Government Expands Scope of Attack on Licenses of Wisconsin Foundation

Special to THE NEW YORK TIMES.. **New York Times (1857-Current file).** New York, N.Y.: Oct 21, 1944. pg. 7, 1 pgs

Abstract (Document Summary)

CHICAGO, Oct. 20 -- The scope of *the Government's anti-trust suit attacking the legality of the licensing system under which the Wisconsin Alumni Research Foundation handles its vitamin D process patents was enlarged today with the naming of 17 more defendants,* one individual and 16 food and medicinal products companies.

Comment: It therefore appears that the subject of patent control of vitamins in 1944 was a very hot subject in the courts and in the press.

Oct 22, 1944
Quantity Production of Vitamins

W.K.. **New York Times (1857-Current file).** New York, N.Y.: Oct 22, 1944. pg. E9, 1 pgs

Abstract (Document Summary)

Fifteen years ago Dr. Kenneth C.D. Hickman of Rochester, N.Y., began to experiment with high vacuums to dry photographic film for tropical shipment. Now he is using the same method to wring vitamins out of raw materials. *Out of his work, an industry has grown which is now the largest producer of vitamin A concentrates and the only large-scale producer of vitamin B.*

Comment: Thus in 1944 medical researchers were spending a lot of time and money to perfect the manufacture of vitamins.

May 17, 1945
B COMPLEX IS USED IN DIABETES CASES; Two Doctors Report Need for Insulin Reduced or Even Ended by Treatment

New York Times (1857-Current file). New York, N.Y.: May 17, 1945. pg. 14, 1 pgs

Abstract (Document Summary)

The use of *vitamin B complex in the treatment of diabetes, resulting in a reduction in insulin requirement and sometimes its elimination, or a reduction in insulin reaction*, was described last night at the New York Academy of Medicine in a paper presented by Dr. Morton S. Biskind and Dr. Herbert Schreier. It was one of ...

Comment: It therefore appears that, medical researchers in 1945 were determining that yet another vitamin, vitamin-B, is capable of helping diabetics to reduce insulin. If such a drug were produced, it would have been worth billions of dollars. Meanwhile the FDA continues to suppress claims made on vitamins.

Jan 15, 1946
VITAMIN D PATENTS GIVEN TO THE PUBLIC; U.S. Court Decree Ends Civil Anti-Trust Suit Against Wisconsin Foundation
PROHIBITIVE COST' CITED Asst. Dist. Attorney Says Persons Who Most Needed Rickets Cure Were Unable to Get It

Special to THE NEW YORK TIMES.. **New York Times (1857-Current file).** New York, N.Y.: Jan 15, 1946. pg. 16, 1 pgs

Abstract (Document Summary)

CHICAGO, Jan. 14--*Patents controlling Vitamin D, the so called "Sunshine Vitamin," which prevents and cures rickets, became public property today* when Federal Judge John P. Barnes signed a consent judgment terminating a civil anti-trust suit filed last October against the Wisconsin Alumni Foundation and seventeen other defendants.

Comment: The basic law of patenting is that no one can patent a natural substance, and since all vitamins were made by God, then no one should ever have been allowed a patent, although up to this time, several were granted.

Apr 9, 1947

Expert Urges Doubling Our Consumption of Vitamin A Through Foods Rich in It

By *JANE NICKERSON*. **New York Times (1857-Current File)**. New York, N.Y.: Apr 9, 1947. pg. 28, 1 pgs

Abstract (Document Summary)

After reading about his studies on the vitamin A requirements of whites rats, we called Dr. Henry C. Sherman, Mitchill Professor Emeritus of Chemistry at Columbia University, to inquire further about the significance of his research so far as human beings are concerned.

Comment: It is interesting to note that the United Nations Health Agency reported in 2000 that the lives of one million were saved using vitamin-A supplementation. Apparently Dr. Sherman was a man before his time.

Mar 9, 1949

$72,904,214 SALES SET MERCK RECORD; Profit for '48 Was $8,520,250, or $7.36 a Share, Compared to $5.43 for Year Before

New York Times (1857-Current File). New York, N.Y.: Mar 9, 1949. pg. 41, 1 pgs

Abstract (Document Summary)

Reporting on operations last year of Merck & Co., Inc., drug and chemical concern, George W. Merck, president, *informed shareholders in the report issued for release today that sales were the highest in the company's history* even though price averages for the most important product groups were lower than in 1947.

Comment: $72,904,212 of sales in 1949 is equivalent to $1,690,,000,000 in 2005 dollars, with a genuinely horrific profit of $198,000,000 in 2005 dollars, which, in order to maintain, requires the suppression of vitamin sales. And remember Merck is just one of hundreds of drug companies.

Oct 23, 1949

Diet and Arteries; Tests Show Lack of Vitamin B-6 May Cause Arteriosclerosis

New York Times (1857-Current file). New York, N.Y.: Oct 23, 1949. pg. E9, 1 pgs

Abstract (Document Summary)

Arteries may harden for lack of pyridoxine, vitamin B-6, according to the tentative conclusion reached by Drs. James F. Rinehart and Louis D. Greenberg of the University of California Medical School.

Comment: Thus claims have been made by the University of California which "concluded" that arteries harden for a lack of vitamin-B6. Also in the late 1990s Dr. Kilmer McCulley , Dean of Medicine, University of New York discovered that the hardening of the arteries was caused by an acid buildup, due to mineral deficiency, around the arteries. Vitamin-B6 helps against this acid.

Aug 28, 1965

Research Group Protests

Special to The New York Times. **New York Times (1857-Current file).** New York, N.Y.: Aug 28, 1965. pg. 23, 1 pgs

Abstract (Document Summary)

MADISON, Wis., Aug 27 -- *Restrictions proposed by the Federal Food and Drug Administration on the addition of vitamin D to food products drew a sharp response here today from a spokesman for a university foundation that has been marketing vitamin D for 40 years.*

Comment: Therefore, 21 years after being defeated by Congress for attempting to control vitamins by making them a drug, the FDA , in 1965 chose to prevent the use of vitamin-D in food. This is ironic because putting a food, vitamin-D into another food is a natural and safe thing to do. The real concern of the FDA is that by allowing this practice to continue, the medical claims of improved health will become more prominent in the press.

Dec 14, 1972

Drug Agency Acts to Restrict Use of Diet Pills and Vitamins; DRUG AGENCY ACTS FOR CURB ON PILLS

By RICHARD D. LYONS Special to The New York Times. **New York Times (1857-Current file)**. New York, N.Y.: Dec 14, 1972. pg. 97, 2 pgs

Abstract (Document Summary)

WASHINGTON, Dec. 13 -- *The Food and Drug Administration announced moves today to restrict unnecessary and potentially harmful use of diet pills and vitamins.*

Comment: The FDA had no proof of the harm of vitamins, so they resort to taking action due to "potentially harmful use".

Sep 25, 1973

Superdoses of Vitamins To Be Limited Monday

New York Times (1857-Current file). New York, N.Y.: Sep 25, 1973. pg. 12, 1 pgs

Abstract (Document Summary)

Barring last- minute court intervention, *this is the last week that Americans will be able to buy high-concentration doses of vitamin A or vitamin D without a prescription.*

Comment: The question to be asked is that if high doses of vitamin-A or D were harmful (note hundreds of scientific studies had proven this not to be true) then why was the drug industry allowed to sell them by subscriptions. Logic says that if it were toxic that buying it from a doctor would cause the same harm as buying it from a store.

Oct 1, 1973
OUTPUT OF VITAMINS UNDER RESTRICTIONS
New York Times (1857-Current file). New York, N.Y.: Oct 1, 1973. pg. 30, 1 pgs

Abstract (Document Summary)

Further production of super-strength Vitamin A and D products labeled for nonprescription use is barred by new Federal regulations taking effect at midnight.

Health Food Groups to Sue Over Vitamins A and D Curb
New York Times (1857-Current file). New York, N.Y.: Oct 2, 1973. pg. 22, 1 pgs

Abstract (Document Summary)

Two health food organizations announced today that they would go to court to try to stop the Food and Drug Administration from banning the sales of large doses of Vitamins A and D without a prescription.

Comment: Thus the legal battle continues between the drug industry trying to eliminate vitamins and those believing the merits to good health by the use of vitamins, which includes the bulk of the American scientific community.

Oct 26, 1973
Linus Pauling to Challenge F.D.A.'s Curb on Vitamins
New York Times (1857-Current file). New York, N.Y.: Oct 26, 1973. pg. 87, 1 pgs

Abstract (Document Summary)

Dr. Linus Pauling, twice winner of the Nobel Prize, said today he would go to court to try to stop the Food and Drug Administration from imposing its new controls on vitamins.

Comment: The FDA would soon find that an advocate like Linus Pauling could and would present difficult obstacles to their anti-vitamin programs.

Aug 15, 1974
F.D.A. VITAMIN CURBS SCORED BY PROXMIRE
New York Times (1857-Current file). New York, N.Y.: Aug 15, 1974. pg. 34, 1 pgs

Abstract (Document Summary)

Senator William Proxmire, Democrat of Wisconsin accused the Food and Drug Administration today of trying to assume too much power with proposed controls over vitamins. The agency in turn predicted there would be widespread consumer fraud and unchecked quackery unless its new regulations went into effect on the first of next year as scheduled.

Comment: Ironically, some of the most prestigious men the world has ever known, including Albert Einstein, were once called quacks by their contemporaries. The use of name calling, ie: quack, only occurs when no logical arguments can be given. The FDA is referring to the thousands of scientist who claim health benefits from vitamins. It should also be noted that before the 1994 Health Act was created giving total freedom to dispense vitamins to the supplement industry, Congress voted several times against the FDA actions and also their never was any consumer fraud or unchecked quackery.

Sep 19, 1974
F.D.A. CHIEF BACKS RULES FOR VITAMINS
New York Times (1857-Current file). New York, N.Y.: Sep 19, 1974. pg. 36, 1 pgs

Abstract (Document Summary)

Congress should keep its hands off the Food and Drug Administration's plans to regulate the vitamin industry, Alexander M. Schmidt, the Commissioner of Food and Drugs, said today.

Comment: Of course the FDA does not want Congress who represent the people to have a say as the people have already spoken against the FDA plans.

Sep 29, 1974
Votes in Congress; House Senate Last Week's Tally for Metropolitan Area

New York Times (1857-Current file). New York, N.Y.: Sep 29, 1974. pg. 57, 1 pgs

Abstract (Document Summary)

1. *Vote on amendment providing that Food and Drug Administration regulate vitamins as foods and not as drugs, which passed, 81 to 10, Sept. 24*. 2. Vote on Health Professions Educational Assistance Act, which passed, 81 to 7, Sept. 24.

Comment: It therefore appears that the FDA did not get its way by claiming that vitamins were drugs. They were over-ruled by the people.

May 28, 1975

F.D.A. EASES RULES ON SOME VITAMINS; Agency Changes '73 Decision to Control Them as Drugs *A and D Still Curbed*

By DAVID BURNHAM Special to The New York Times. **New York Times (1857-Current file)**. New York, N.Y.: May 28, 1975. pg. 85, 2 pgs

Abstract (Document Summary)

WASHINGTON, May 27 *The Food and Drug Administration backed away today from its decision of 1973 that super potent vitamins and minerals should be regulated as drugs.*

Comment: This is ironic as the drug industry made the "super potent" vitamin-D into best selling drugs, even though they were basically the food supplement called vitamins.

Apr 14, 1976
Congress Blocks Efforts by F.D.A. To Curb Vitamins

New York Times (1857-Current file). New York, N.Y.: Apr 14, 1976. pg. 16, 1 pgs

Abstract (Document Summary)

Congress has passed a bill blocking the Food and Drug Administration's attempts to regulate the sale of high-potency vitamin and mineral pills.

Comment: Once again the peoples representatives speak out against the puppets of the drug industry, the FDA.

Sep 26, 1977
RULES FOR PRESCRIPTION ON SOME VITAMINS

ENDED

New York Times (1857-Current file). New York, N.Y.: Sep 26, 1977. pg. 36, 1 pgs

Abstract (Document Summary)

WASHINGTON, Sept. 25 (UPI) *After four years of public dispute and court battles, the Government has dropped its attempt to require a doctor's prescription for high potency doses of vitamins A and D.* The health food industry, which had fought the Government, *hailed the decision as a victory for consumer freedom of choice.*

Comment: Amen !!!

Mar 16, 1978

F.D.A. Revokes Rules to Restrict Large Doses of Vitamins A and D

New York Times (1857-Current file). New York, N.Y.: Mar 16, 1978. pg. B14, 1 pgs

Abstract (Document Summary)

WASHINGTON, March 15 (UPI)--*The Food and Drug Administration has revoked rules first proposed more than five years ago in an attempt to make large doses of Vitamins A and D available only with a doctor's prescription.*

Comment: The FDA was beaten but not down as it would continue its propaganda campaign against vitamins. (see Mar 12, 1979 report)

Mar 12, 1979

F.D.A Panel Urges Curb On Some Vitamin Sales

New York Times (1857-Current file). New York, N.Y.: Mar 12, 1979. pg. B9, 1 pgs

Abstract (Document Summary)

WASHINGTON, March 11 (AP)--*A Government advisory panel recommended today that curbs be imposed on sales of some vitamins and minerals as nonprescription drugs* and that labels mentioning "super potency," "natural" or "stress" be banned.

Comment: Once again the FDA is trying to impose the will of the drug industry on the people.

Feb 26, 1980
Vitamin D Used to Treat Bone Disease; Vitamin D Used in Bone Disease

By JANE E. BRODY. **New York Times (1857-Current file)**. New York, N.Y.: Feb 26, 1980. pg. C1, 2 pgs

Abstract (Document Summary)

WHAT began 15 years ago as basic research into the workings of vitamin D has produced unexpected dividends for the treatment of several human diseases, including possibly osteoporosis, the bone-thinning disorder that afflicts millions of older Americans.

Vitamin-D now has another prestigious medical claim that the FDA will try to cover up.

Nov 29, 1985
Calcium in Diet May Cut Risk Of Colon Cancer, Study Finds

New York Times (1857-Current file). New York, N.Y.: Nov 29, 1985. pg. B20, 1 pgs

Abstract (Document Summary)

BOSTON, Nov. 28 (AP) -- *A new study provides biological evidence supporting the theory that people may be able to lower the risk of colon cancer by adding calcium to the diet,* according to an article published today.

Comment: As vitamin-D is the biological partner of calcium, then vitamin-D also helps to prevent colon cancer as hundreds of other researchers in the future would prove to be true.

Dec 6, 1990

Sunlight and Breast Cancer: Danger in Darkness?

By NATALIE ANGIER. **New York Times (1857-Current file).** New York, N.Y.: Dec 6, 1990. pg. B18, 1 pgs

Abstract (Document Summary)

Women who live in northern cities where towering buildings block what feeble winter sun there is may have a higher risk of breast cancer than women in southern regions where sunlight abounds, a new study suggests.

Comment: This study implies that vitamin-D from the sun prevents breast cancer. The FDA must be squirming.

Dec 12, 1990

Doctors Given Millions by Drug Companies

By WARREN E. LEARY Special to The New York Times. **New York Times (1857-Current file).** New York, N.Y.: Dec 12, 1990. pg. B13, 1 pgs

Abstract (Document Summary)

WASHINGTON, Dec. 11 -- *A Senate survey made public today said drug companies were spending more than $165 million a year on gifts, trips and payments for doctors in hopes of influencing their prescription decisions.*

Comment: Obviously none of these doctors will prescribe life sustaining vitamins to their patients.

May 26, 1991
Black People Need Vitamin D Supplements
JOEL D. SCHIFF. **New York Times (1857-Current file)**. New York, N.Y.: May 26, 1991. pg. LI17, 1 pgs

Abstract (Document Summary)

The report of increasing incidence of osteoporosis among black women ["Why Is Osteoporosis Rising for Blacks?" April 14] should not come as a surprise. Bone mass and the calcification of bone are normally maintained by adequate levels of vitamin D, which is both a hormone and a nutrient.

Comment: Vitamin-D is thus proven to be of great value to Blacks with osteoporosis.

Jan 29, 1992
Profits Rise 19.8% at Merck
By MILT FREUDENHEIM. **New York Times (1857-Current file)**. New York, N.Y.: Jan 29, 1992. pg. D4, 1 pgs

Abstract (Document Summary)

Merck & Company added to its string of double-digit earnings gains in the final quarter of 1991.

And they made much of these profits selling lethal drugs to people who were desperate for vitamins.

Feb 6, 1992
Study Finds Vitamin Counters Osteoporosis
New York Times (1857-Current file). New York, N.Y.: Feb 6, 1992. pg. B7, 1 pgs

ABSRACT BOSTON, Feb. 5 (AP) -- *A synthetic form of vitamin D appears to reduce the risk of fractures significantly in older women with brittle bones, a new study has found.*

Comment: This study reflects hundreds of other studies concluding the same thing.

May 16, 1992
A Variation Of Vitamin D Aids Bones
Edmund L. Andrews. **New York Times (1857-Current file).** New York, N.Y.: May 16, 1992. pg. 41, 1 pgs

Abstract (Document Summary)

WASHINGTON MOTHERS and nutritionists have said for decades that drinking milk, rich in calcium and fortified with vitamin D, can help build strong bones and teeth in growing children.

Comment: The expression that "Mother knows best" is quite appropriate.

Aug 9, 1992
F.D.A. Steps Up Effort to Control Vitamin Claims; F.D.A. Acts to Control Vitamin Claims

By *LENA WILLIAMS*. **New York Times (1857-Current file)**. New York, N.Y.: Aug 9, 1992. pg. 1, 2 pgs

Abstract (Document Summary)

In Texas, *state health inspectors raided health food stores across the state in May and, as startled customers and bystanders watched in amazement, removed hundreds of products, including vitamin C, aloe vera products and herbal teas.*

Comment: The FDA has declared war on the American people.

Sep 8, 1992
Yes, F.D.A. Wants to Block Sale of Vitamins

BERNARD RIMLAND. **New York Times (1857-Current file)**. New York, N.Y.: Sep 8, 1992. pg. A18, 1 pgs

Abstract (Document Summary)

I am one of the millions of Americans outraged by the Food and Drug Administration's unwarranted efforts to keep me from purchasing the nutritional supplements I desire (front page, Aug. 9). My outrage is in no way mitigated by the unconvincing protestations of innocence and good intentions of David A. Kessler, the F.D.A. Commissioner, in your Aug. 16 "correction" article.

Comment: Apparently the FDA will never give up its war on vitamins. What the FDA needs is a nutrient savvy leader.

Jun 15, 1993
F.D.A. Is Again Proposing to Regulate Vitamins and Supplements

By *MARIAN BURROS Special to The New York Times*. **New York Times (1857-Current file)**. New York, N.Y.: Jun 15,

1993. pg. A25, 1 pgs

Abstract (Document Summary)

WASHINGTON, June 14 -- *The Food and Drug Administration will renew its efforts to control vitamins and other dietary supplements on Tuesday, when it announces plans to regulate health claims.* The agency will also seek advice on how to assure the safety of the products in the $4 billion market.

Comment: **The FDA's efforts to destroy the vitamin market will never end.**

Mar 7, 1994

U.S. DRUG INDUSTRY FIGHTS REPUTATION FOR PRICE GOUGING: *Pharmaceutical Makers Focus Energies on Advertising and Target Key Legislators U.S.*

By NEIL A. LEWIS with ROBERT PEAR Special to The New York Times. **New York Times (1857-Current file).** New York, N.Y.: Mar 7, 1994. pg. A1, 2 pgs

Abstract (Document Summary)

WASHINGTON, March 6 -- *When President Clinton stood before an audience at an Arlington, Va., health clinic last year and characterized the pharmaceutical industry as a bunch of price gougers,* executives of the nation's drug companies had what their scientists might call a convulsive reaction.

Comment: **The average increase from the cost of the ingredients of the following 16 drug to the consumer price was 79,000 %, or the drugs sell for almost 800 times cost of their ingredients. WOW !!!**

Was President Clinton wrong?
The chart below speaks for itself.

Celebrex:100mg

Consumer price (100 tablets): $130.27

Cost of active ingredients: $0.60

Percent markup:

21,712%

Prozac:20mg

Consumer price (100 tablets) : $247.47

Cost of active ingredients: $0.11

Percent markup:

224,973% (WOW !!!)

Claritin:10mg

Consumer Price (100 tablets): $215.17

Cost of active ingredients: $0.71

Percent markup:

30,306%

Tenormin:50mg

Consumer price (100 tablets): $104.47

Cost of active ingredients: $0.13

Percent markup:

80,362%

Keflex:250mg

Consumer Price (100 tablets): $157.39

Cost of active ingredients:

Vasotec:10mg

Consumer price (100 tablets): $10237

Cost of active ingredients:

$1.88

Percent markup:

8,372%

$0.20

Percent markup:

51,185%

Lipitor:20 mg

Consumer Price (100 tablets): $272.37

Cost of active ingredients: $5.80

Percent markup:

4,696%

Xanax:1mg

Consumer price (100 tablets) : $136.79

Cost of active ingredients: $0.024

Percent markup:

569,958%

Norvasec:10mg

Consumer price (100 tablets): $188.29

Cost of active ingredients: $0.14

Percent markup:

134,493%

Zestril:20mg

Consumer price (100 tablets) $89.89

Cost of active ingredients: $3.20

Percent markup:

2,809%

Paxil:20mg

Consumer price (100 tablets): $220.27

Cost of active ingredients: $7.60

Percent markup:

<u>2,898%</u>

Prevacid:30mg

Consumer price (100 tablets): $44.77

Cost of active ingredients: $1.01

Percent markup:

<u>34,136%</u>

Prilosec:20mg

Consumer price (100 tablets): $360.97

Cost of active ingredients:

Zithromax:600mg

Consumer price (100 tablets): $1,482.19

Cost of active ingredients: $18.78

Percent markup:

<u>7,892%</u>

Zocor:40mg

Consumer price (100 tablets): $350.27

Cost of active ingredients: $8.63

Percent markup:

<u>4,059%</u>

Zoloft:50mg

Consumer price: $206.87

Cost of active ingredients:

$0.52 $1.75

Percent markup: Percent markup:

69,417%   11,821%

Budget Analyst, US Department of Commerce

Mar 12, 1995

Rickets, a Relic, Shows Up Again; Breast-fed infants have been getting a rare bone disease. Rickets, a Disease That All But Vanished, Shows Up Again Rickets' return can reflect parents' confusion and their financial concerns.

By KAREN TORTORELLA. **New York Times (1857-Current file).** New York, N.Y.: Mar 12, 1995. pg. NJ1, 2 pgs

Abstract (Document Summary)

FOR generations, the bone disease called rickets has been virtually nonexistent in America. The addition of vitamin D to milk, which began in the 1930's, all but eliminated what was a major health hazard for young children.

Comment: The truth is that the small amount of vitamin-D in milk is not enough for good health.

Aug 9, 1995

Vitamin A and Infants With H.I.V.

New York Times (1857-Current file). New York, N.Y.: Aug 9, 1995. pg. C8, 1 pgs

Abstract (Document Summary)

WASHINGTON, Aug. 8 (AP) -- *Vitamin A might be an inexpensive way to ease some of the illnesses suffered by infants with the AIDS virus, new research suggests.*

Comment: Another gold star for a crucial vitamin.

May, 2005
Vitamin-D Research Turning Sunscreen Wisdom on Head,
Phoenix Arizona Republic, May 22, 2005

Abstract: *"I would challenge anyone to find an area or nutrient or any factor that has such consistent anti-cancer benefits as vitamin-D."* The thinking is that even if too much sun leads to the non lethal skin cancer, too little sun may be worse.. *"I find the evidence that the sun prevents cancer to be mountingnd increasingly compelling* (Dr. AllenHaloern, dermatology chief at Memorial Sloan-Kettering Cancer Center, New York.)

Comment: Obviously the cancer researchers in 2005 are emphatic in their belief that vitamin-D cures cancer.

SUMMARY
Of Newspaper Articles

If the preceding newspaper articles are a reflection of the truth, then the true story is that we now have the technology and understanding of human health which will allow us to wipe out degenerative diseases. And remember that today's newspapers are full of hundreds of stories that support this view. From the very beginning, at the turn of the last century, these newspaper stories demonstrated that the

153

scientific community believed that vitamins prolong life and inhibit disease. Also from the very beginning, these same newspaper stories have showed that all government agencies have been trying to suppress this information, while controlling the sale of the vitamins to the exclusion of all others. Over the past 80 years, despite being admonished by the courts and Congress, government agencies still refuse to abide by the law. Their message is constant. *They want control of the sale of vitamins for the benefit of the drug industry, which, because vitamins work to suppress disease, they want to package them as drugs.* The newspaper stories demonstrate just how important vitamins have been to society since their discovery 95 years ago, and how much money has been spent trying to promote, patent, exploit and suppress these vitamins. Vitamins were definitely one of the top stories of the last century, and when we finally use them to wipe out disease, and we will, vitamins and God's other nutrients will become the top story of this century.

However, when we use the knowledge of vitamins and minerals to wipe out disease, this will result in massive financial loses for the most powerful and the most profitable drug industry whose boards of directors are lined with individuals that once represented government agencies that were supposed to represent the people. The Food and Drug Administration, FDA, the Federal Trade Commission, FTC, and the American Medical Association, AMA, all have demonstrated that that they want to control the vitamin industry for the benefit of the drug industry. The FDA refuses to exercise its mandate and evaluate the medical merits of food, because food cannot be patented and therefore, the drug industry would be financially harmed. Dr Reich used to say that FDA stands for Food Dis-information Agency. It is obvious that FDA is a misnomer and they should take the word "food" out of their name and just be called what they are, the Drug Agency., the DA.

At the turn of the last century, cancer was at 3%. Then, 50 years later in 1950 cancer was at 20% and all of the government agencies were scrambling to find a drug that worked, in spite of the scientific evidence reported in the newspaper articles that vitamin and minerals were working. Then, only fifty years later in 2000 cancer was at 40%, one out of four people have mental disorders and one out of eight have diabetes. Meanwhile the government agencies are still scrambling to find their first drug that would work, despite the massive scientific evidence of the day that showed vitamins and minerals worked and the fact that they have made it against the law for the public to make medical claims on vitamins. Today, they are still scrambling to find a drug and they are still attempting to suppress the use of vitamins and minerals that have been proven to work. Its unfortunate, but the reality is that they will never find their drug and if society waits much longer for these idiots, we may not survive as a species.

This tragedy is compounded by the fact that Black America dies six years before White America and has over twice the degenerative diseases. The simple question becomes, "If white America died six years before Black America and was twice as sick as Black America, would these same government agencies spend money to find out why???" I personally believe they would spend hundreds of billions of dollars, maybe trillions. If you believe this to be true, then you must ask yourself, why haven't they spent any money on Black America? Not one nickel!

There can only be one answer, and that is racial prejudice of the worst kind that has resulted in the premature and painful deaths of millions of Black Americans. Remember *that two time Nobel Prize winner, Otto Warburg M.D. warned Americans in 1966* that because of these agnostic government agencies, *"millions of people would die needlessly form cancer."* Unfortunately his prediction has come true and the man responsible for these government agencies, that are currently perpetrating the worst form of racial prejudice in the history of America, is the leaders of our government & the President of the United States. *Where is our President when the people need him most???* I believe all Americans, especially Black Americans, should be emotionally lobbying the President to take action against this injustice that should make all Americans ashamed. I personally am heartbroken and I just want to scream !!!

CHAPTER ELEVEN

THE HUMAN NEED FOR

SUN ON THE SKIN

In 1982, when I realized that Dr. Reich had been curing diseases using calcium nutrition and the sunshine vitamin, vitamin-D, I began to realize as a biochemist just how potent vitamin-D was against disease. Logically, hundreds of functions occur when the sun strikes living things. Plants could not survive without the sunshine nor could humans. And yet, the men of medicine are adamant that the sun causes diseases and should be avoided at all cost. *This is not very logical as the sun striking the human body initiates hundreds of biological functions,* all of which are necessary for survival of the human race. *God placed the pituitary, pineal and hypo thymus glands directly behind the eyes* where they could be exposed to direct sunlight. *When UV light strikes these glands, they cause the body to produce a host of hormones, like calcitonin, serotonin and melatonin, and enzymes, like inisotol triphosphate, that are crucial for life.* However, the most crucial function is the production of vitamin-D from cholesterol in the skin. Therefore, exposure to sunlight is crucial for human survival.

157

Despite this, the *men of medicine declare that God made a mistake when he made the sun* as they believe that "the sun causes cancer". Of course, I have been lecturing the opposite since 1982, and the men of medicine have belittled my efforts and suggested that my actions were criminal. Today, the tide is shifting as hundreds of our best medical scientists are declaring that the sun prevents a host of diseases. The subject is being discussed in newspapers and on television. However, because of decades of brainwashing, these scientists and the public are still reluctant to open the door to sunbathing. Despite this, the cultures all over the world that are virtually disease free spend many hours in the sun each day and finally some of our best medical scientists are now extolling the virtues of sun on the skin. For example, WB Grant in his publication *"Ecologic studies of solar UV-B radiation and cancer mortality rates"* writes, *"Solar ultraviolet B (UV-B) radiation (280-320 nm) has been associated with reduced risk of cancer of the breast, colon, ovary, and prostate, as well as non-Hodgkin's lymphoma (NHL) through the production of vitamin D and has been written about in papers extending back to 1980. Using data on the geographic distribution of cancer mortality rates in the US, another ten cancers have been added to the list for which UV-B/vitamin D is a risk reduction factor (Grant 2002b; submitted").*

Grant further states that these associations persist even after additional cancer risk and risk reduction factors such as smoking, urban or rural residence, Hispanic heritage, poverty, dietary factors, and use of non-steroidal anti-inflammatory drugs are added to the analysis. *Inverse correlations are found for UV-B radiation for a number of* *cancers, with those for bladder, breast, endometrial, ovarian, prostate, and renal cancer, and multiple melanoma and NHL* having the strongest correlations in this and ongoing multi-country ecologic studies.

These studies add further support for the role of UV-B radiation and vitamin D in reducing the risk of a large number of cancers. PMID: 12899536 [PubMed - indexed for MEDLINE]

Other scientists have found that sunlight is specifically effective at reducing specific cancers For example, C.L. Hanchette and G.G. Schwartz of the Department of Geography, University of North Carolina, Chapel Hill in their scientific publication *"Geographic patterns of prostate cancer mortality.* Evidence for a protective effect of ultraviolet radiation" concluded that their data lend support to the hypothesis that *"UV radiation may protect against clinical prostate cancer".*
PMID: 1451068 [PubMed - indexed for MEDLINE]

Also, viewed in conjunction with other recent data, including those demonstrating a differentiating effect of vitamin D on human prostate cancer cells, the authors found that *"these findings suggest that vitamin D may have an important role in the natural history of prostate cancer."*

It should be noted that Prostate cancer is the **most prevalent non-skin cancer among men in the United States and is** *the second leading cause of cancer deaths in men.*

Because the major source of vitamin D is casual exposure to ultraviolet (UV) radiation, the authors examined the *geographic distributions of UV radiation and prostate cancer mortality in 3073 counties of the contiguous United States* using linear regression and trend surface analyses. The results were conclusive: the <u>*geographic distributions of UV radiation and prostate cancer mortality are correlated inversely and prostate cancer mortality exhibits a significant north-south trend, with lower rates in the South.*</u> These geographic patterns are not readily explicable by other known risk factors for prostate cancer.

Hanchette and Swartz are joined by Chen TC Holick of the Vitamin D, Skin and Bone Research Laboratory, Section of Endocrinology, Diabetes and Nutrition, Department of Medicine, Boston University School of Medicine, Boston, MA 02118, USA, who in his publication *"Vitamin D and prostate cancer prevention and treatment"*, states *"that human prostate cells contain receptors for vitamin-D and the prostate cancer cells respond to vitamin D(3) with increases in differentiation and apoptosis, and decreases in proliferation, invasiveness and metastasis"* and that *"these findings strongly support the use of vitamin D-based therapies for prostate cancer".* Holick further states that *"the association between either decreased sun exposure or vitamin D deficiency and the increased risk of prostate cancer at an earlier age, and with a more aggressive progression, indicates that* ***adequate vitamin D nutrition should be a priority for men of all ages.*** PMID: 14580762 [PubMed - indexed for MEDLINE]

Then, adding another degenerative disease to the list of diseases that can be cured by vitamin-D, C.E Hayes, M.T. Cantorna and H.F. DeLuca of the Department of Biochemistry, University of Wisconsin-Madison 53706, USA writes in their publication *"Vitamin-D and Multiple Sclerosis"* that *"Recently, it has been clearly demonstrated that **the hormonal form of vitamin D3, can completely prevent experimental autoimmune encephalomyelitis (EAE), a widely accepted mouse model of human multiple sclerosis (MS).** This finding has focused attention on the possible relationship of this disease to vitamin D".*

In addition they further write that *"It is our hypothesis that one crucial environmental factor is the degree of sunlight exposure catalyzing the **production of vitamin D3 in skin, and, further, that the hormonal form of vitamin D3 is a selective immune system regulator inhibiting this autoimmune disease.** Therefore, under low-sunlight conditions, **insufficient vitamin D3 is produced, limiting production of vitamin D3, providing a risk for MS.***

The authors note that *"This theory can explain the striking geographic distribution **of MS, which is nearly zero in equatorial regions and increases dramatically with latitude in both hemispheres and it can also explain two peculiar geographic anomalies, one in <u>Switzerland</u> with high MS rates at low altitudes and low MS rates at high altitudes, and one in <u>Norway</u> with a high MS prevalence inland and a lower MS prevalence along the coast".***

The authors reasoned that *Ultraviolet (UV) light intensity is higher at high altitudes, resulting in a greater vitamin D3 synthetic rate,* thereby accounting for low MS rates at higher altitudes. On the <u>Norwegian coast</u>, *fish is consumed at high rates and fish oils are rich in vitamin- D3.*

Also, further, *experimental work on EAE provides strong support for the importance of vitamin D3 in reducing the risk and susceptibility for MS.* Therefore, vitamin-D3 or its analogs may have great therapeutic potential in patients with MS. More importantly, current research together with data from migration studies opens the possibility that *MS may be preventable in genetically susceptible individuals with early intervention strategies that provide adequate levels of hormonally active vitamin-D3 or its analogs.*
PMID: 9316607 [PubMed - indexed for MEDLINE]

All of the previously mentioned researchers claiming vitamin-D cures have been joined by John EM, Schwartz GG, Dreon DM, Koo J. of the Northern California Cancer Center, Union City 94587, USA, who in their publication "Vitamin D and breast cancer risk: the NHANES I Epidemiologic follow-up study, 1971-1975 to 1992. National Health and Nutrition Examination survey", write that *"By analyzing data from the first National Health and Nutrition Examination Survey Epidemiologic Follow-up Study to test the hypothesis that vitamin D from sunlight exposure, diet, and supplements reduces the risk of breast cancer, we determined that several measures of sunlight exposure and dietary vitamin D intake were associated with reduced risk of breast cancer, with RRs ranging from 0.67-0.85".*

The study identified 190 women with incident breast cancer from a cohort of 5009 white women who completed the dermatological examination and 24-hour dietary recall conducted from 1971-1974 and who were followed up to 1992. Using Cox proportional hazards regression, relative risks (RRs) were estimated for   breast cancer and 95% confidence intervals, adjusting for age, education, age at menarche, age at menopause, body mass index, alcohol consumption, and physical activity. The associations with vitamin D exposures, however, varied by region of residence. *The risk reductions were highest for women who lived in United States regions of high solar radiation,* with RRs ranging from 0.35-0.75. *No reductions in risk were found for women who lived in regions of low solar radiation.* Although limited by the relatively small size of the case population, the protective effects of vitamin D observed in this prospective study are consistent for several independent measures of vitamin D. *"These data support the hypothesis that <u>sunlight and dietary vitamin D reduce the risk of breast cancer"</u>.*
PMID: 10350434 [PubMed - indexed for MEDLINE]

Finally, the world wide leader, and my hero, in the scientific study of vitamin-D and disease, Dr. Reinhold Vieth from the Department of Laboratory Medicine and Pathobiology, University of Toronto, and Pathology and Laboratory Medicine, Mount Sinai Hospital, Toronto, provides a list of 135 scientific publications in the American Journal of Clinical Nutrition, Vol. 69, No. 5, 842-856, May 1999. These scientific references support his views that sunshine is essential for proper health. **(First page of these references is given next)**

1. Heaney RP. Calcium and vitamin D in human nutrition. In: Lipkin M, Newmark HL, Kelloff GJ, eds. Calcium, vitamin D, and prevention of colon cancer. Boca Raton, FL: CRC Press, 1991:9–10.

2. Takeuchi A, Okano T, Ishida Y, Kobayashi T. Effects of dietary vitamin D intake on plasma levels of parathyroid hormone and vitamin D metabolites in healthy Japanese. Miner Electrolyte Metab 1995;21:217–22.[Medline]

3. National Academy of Sciences. Recommended dietary allowances. 10th ed. Washington, DC: National Academy Press, 1989.

4. Park EA. The therapy of rickets. JAMA 1940;115:370–9.

5. Blumberg RW, Forbes GB, Fraser D, et al. The prophylactic requirement and the toxicity of vitamin D. Pediatrics 1963;31:512–25.[Abstract]

6. Smith R, Dent CE. Vitamin D requirements in adults. Clinical and metabolic studies on seven patients with nutritional osteomalacia. Bibl Nutr Dieta 1969;13:44–5.[Medline]

7. Parfitt AM, Gallagher JC, Heaney RP, Johnston CC, Neer R, Whedon GD. Vitamin D and bone health in the elderly. Am J Clin Nutr 1982;36:1014–31.[Abstract]

8. Utiger RD. The need for more vitamin D. N Engl J Med 1998;338:828–9.[Free Full Text]

9. Thomas MK, Lloyd-Jones DM, Thadhani RI, et al. Hypovitaminosis D in medical inpatients. N Engl J Med 1998;338:777–83.[Abstract/Free Full Text]

CHAPTER TWELVE

VITAMIN-D AND BLACK AMERICA

Every once in a while the newspaper will write an article on just how sick Black America is with a specific particular disease. When all of the articles are collected, however, a much different story appears. Black America suffers from highest cancer rates of all ethnic groups, (**American Cancer Society:** *"Cancer Facts and Figures for African Americans 2004-2005", Blacks have approximately 30 to 40% more cancer and in some cases a 250% higher death rate than Whites) twice the diabetes and five times the kidney disease.*

And even more tragically, *life expectancy for Black men is 68.6 years old* compared to 75.0 for White men(**6.4 year difference**) and *Black women are 75.5* versus 80.2 for White women **(4.7Year Difference)** (**American Cancer Society,** *"Cancer Facts and Figures for African Americans 2004-2005).* This is a *"six year discrepancy"* for men and almost a *five year discrepancy* for women that makes me want to scream!!! I am very angry that the medical authorities can stand by and let this happen. In my life, I have never seen a worse form of racial prejudice. It makes me sick and ashamed to live in America. *It is definitely the crime of the century.* Black America is dramatically sicker than White America and dying much younger. **Why???   Why??? Why???   Why???**   Please, Oprah Winfrey, Jesse Jackson and Willy Cooper, help me stop this injustice !!!

And why don't the medical authorities do something about this absolutely disgraceful situation? And, why don't White Americans even know about it? And why aren't the Blacks talking about it? Unfortunately, the answers lie in our ignorance and the medical authorities who are leading us. *In 100 years of trying they have not been able to inhibit or cure even one disease, not one!!!* These generals of medicine have been leading us in a war against disease where they have lost every battle. And then, when they win a little skirmish, they make sure that they get credit and it is given front page headlines. The reason that they are loosing this war, where all of our lives are dependant, including those of our children, is that they are looking for a white chemical drug to answer their prayers. This is just never going to happen.

If we are to survive as a nation, or even survive as a species, *we must replace these ignorant generals of medicine in the AMA, FDA and FTC with the men of vision who understand that the answer lies in nutrition.* If I were given charge of these organizations, I would fire the incompetent generals and revamp these organizations to make them serve the public, which is what Congress intended when it created them. There would be dozens of FDA approved medical claims for calcium and vitamin-D and the FTC would stop harassing nutritionists who would now be FDA approved. The FDA would actually assess food and preventive medicine though nutrition which would then become the medicine of the 21st Century. *"If the doctors of today do not become the nutritionists of tomorrow then the nutritionists of today will become the doctors of tomorrow."* ---Rockefeller Institute of Medical Research, New York.

T herefore, there is hope on the horizon, as medical researchers all over the world are finding that supplementation with the humble mineral calcium along with vitamin-D can help to prevent and even cure disease. Thus, *it may soon be possible to cure America, but in fairness, and with Gods help, we must cure Black America first.*

B efore this can happen, we must understand the reason why Black America is so sick. The answer lies on the beaches and at the swimming pools of America, for there you will find Caucasians in bikinis and bathing suits, lapping up the sun and producing vitamin-D, inisitol triphosphate, calcitonin, melitonon, serotonin and a whole bunch of other "tonins". The sun on the skin produces crucial enzymes that regulate mineral disposition in the body. The sun is necessary for good health. While Caucasians flock to these public sun bathing locations, the Black Community avoids the sun like the plague, and in doing so, cuts itself off from its crucial biological functions, such as the production of vitamin-D, and they are thereby being ravaged with disease and dying young.

The sun striking the eyes causes the glands behind them, the pituitary, pineal and hypo thymus to produce the hormones calcitonin, melatonin and serotonin along with others. Therefore, the sun avoiding Black community does not produce these enzymes, hormones and vitamins that are crucial to good health and hence they are twice as sick as the White community. The first step to good health for the Black Community is daily exposure to God's Sunlight and the health benefits that it provides.

.

Unfortunately, there is a further complication with the Black community and the sun. *It is a natural sunscreen called melanin,* that evolved to protect humans from blistering solar radiation as they evolved in equatorial regions of the world. *This skin pigment is an extremely effective sunscreen with absorption properties from the ultraviolet into the visible range. Therefore people of color who have greater amounts of melanin in their epidermis than do whites are less efficient in producing vitamin-D than are whites.* Because of the darkness of there skin and the different content of melanin, Blacks require *10 to 50* times the exposure as whites to produce the same quantity of vitamin-D (*"Vitamin-D: Importance in the Prevention of Cancers, Type 1 Diabetes, Heart Disease, and Osteoporosis"*) *From the Vitamin-D Skin and Bone Research Laboratory, Section of Endocrinology, Diabetes and Nutrition, Department of Medicine, Boston University School of Medicine, Boston MA).* Therefore, *a White man sunbathing for 15 minutes produces more vitamin-D than a Black man sunbathing all day long.* This basically means that regardless of the exposure top sun, Blacks will require vitamin-D supplementation.

Who is usually deficient in Vitamin-D ?

http://my.webmd.com/content/article/78/95751.htm
In the latest study, Gregory A. Plotnikoff, MD, of the University of Minnesota Medical School stated that *all of the African Americans, East Africans, Hispanics, and Native Americans who participated in the study were vitamin-D deficient,* as were all of the patients under the age of 30. The findings are reported in the December 2004 issue of the journal, Mayo Clinic Proceedings.

What diseases have been implicated due to Vitamin D Deficiency?

Alcoholism
Anxiety
Arthritis
Autoimmune diseases
Birth defects
Bone diseases
Bone pain
Burning in mouth
Cancer
Celiac-Sprue
Coeliac
Crohn's
Chronic Fatigue Syndrome
Chronic Pain
Cystic fibrosis
Depression
Diabetes
Diarrhea
Enzymatic diseases
Fatigue

Impaired wound healing
inflammatory bowel disease
Insomnia
Intestine
Irritability
Joint pain
Kidney
Liver
Lupus
Malabsorption
Multiple sclerosis
Muscle pain
Myopia
Nervousness
Obsessive Disorders
Osteomalacea
Osteoporosis
Panic Attacks
Parkinson's
Psoriasis

Fibromyalgia	Rheumatoid arthritis
Graves' disease	Rickets
Heart disease	Scalp sweating
Hernia	Schizophrenia
High blood pressure	Thyroid

*** To review more clinical studies, perform an internet search for "vitamin-D deficiency" and the conditions listed above.

It is also important to note that everyone should avoid wearing glasses as they interfere with light striking the eyes which is crucial for hormone production. Also, avoid skin blocks because they interfere with biological functions. It is highly probable that in the near future there will be multi-billion dollar lawsuits concerning these matters.

Of course, for good health and longevity, a program of calcium and vitamin-D supplementation will be mandatory. Marine coral calcium from Okinawa, Japan is the preferred form of calcium supplementation. *The problem being that most of the coral calcium produced in America is not marine.* It is *fossilized or dirt coral* as it is dug out of the ground and costs a small fraction of the cost of *high grade marine coral harvested from the sea.* Despite this, you will probably be charged high grade prices for the low grade coral and it may even be in a bottle with the Barefoot label. If it is, you will usually be charged less, but you should be aware that the reason for the dirt cheap pricing is because it really is dirt. Unfortunately, surfing on the web for Bob or Robert Barefoot will result in about 2,000,000 hits which means that there is an enormous amount of knock off coral on the market today. If you want to be guaranteed that you are getting the authentic high grade coral calcium endorsed by Barefoot, a phone number will be given on the last page of this book

CHAPTER THIRTEEN

<u>VITAMIN-D SUMMARY</u>

The absorption and utilization of minerals by the human body is dependent on a number of biological and chemical factors, especially the inclusion of vitamin-D in the vitamin-D receptors (VDRs) in the intestine and other organs.

The most important issue is to achieve a regular and optimal intake of major and minor essential minerals that support the chemistry of life, with a major emphasis on calcium. The chemical form in which minerals are presented to the body is a key factor in their efficient utilization in the chemistry of life. Also, the intestine contains about 5000 microbes or bacterium that chew up food, much like a piece of meat left rotting in the sun, and make it amenable for absorption by the body. *The salts produced by the digestive process tend to put this process into hibernation.* The hydrochloric acid in the stomach tends to produce a lot of sodium chloride or salt. However, the injection of marine microbes from coral calcium that thrive in the salts can reactivate the process resulting in a change from relatively low absorption to excellent absorption of the food by the body.

If minerals are presented in a solution in water (in their ionic form), they are used more efficiently in body processes. If coral calcium (basically the mineral aragonite) is added to pure water, a substantial proportion of its valuable contents of minerals becomes ionic, and the marine microbes are liberated. This situation contrasts with minerals like TUMS (calcite or calcium carbonate) taken in dry powder or other supplement forms (e.g. tablets) where less of the minerals may be available for use by the body (bio-available). *The aragonite in coral <u>has over 1000 times the surface area of the calcite in TUMS</u> which accounts for its better dissolution.* Regardless, dissolution in water is irrelevant as within seconds of entering the stomach, over 99% of the coral calcium becomes ionized (test run by Barefoot using stomach acid on coral calcium) and ready for absorption by the body.

During digestion, hydrochloric acid is produced in the stomach and the gastric contents are very acidic, ranging from pH 1 to pH 3. This acid (hydrochloric acid) is produced from the consumption of salt, sodium chloride. Recent studies have shown that doubling the salt intake reduces the production of the hormone, Renin, which results in a dramatic reduction in heart disease as well as prolonging life. Tests have shown that men over 70, who double their salt intake, also double their life span. Contrary to public opinion, no amount of salt has ever raised the blood pressure in any scientific testing. Since almost all minerals containing chlorides are soluble, they remain ionized. The hydrochloric acid secreted by the stomach is a highly effective way of ionizing elements in the food. However, food usually contains products that produce ions other than chlorides, such as the phosphates from meat and soft drinks, the citrates from fruits, and the lactates from milk, to name but a few. It is interesting to note that God made most nutritious foods, such as fruits and vegetables, mildly acidic. They do not have enough acid to effect the level of acid in the stomach, but rather, because of their anions, such as citrates, malates and lactates, they produce strong alkaline salts (such as calcium citrate, calcium malate or calcium lactate) which help to neutralize the acids in the body fluids thereby increasing the oxygen content.

A chelation process occurs to a major degree in coral calcium, according to the chelation therapy expert Dr. Bruce Halstead MD. The act of chelation ("crab claw" binding of metals) is a very important process in nature for the incorporation of vital metals (calcium, magnesium etc.) in body chemistry. Studies have shown that chelated metals are absorbed and used by the body in a more efficient manner than *"plain"* minerals or elements. This is because the chelated mineral has a rod-like form, the perfect shape to penetrate the fingerlike villi which line the small intestine.

In fact, the process of chelation therapy in humans has become a highly valued technique in alternative medicine for removing unwanted metals and treating a variety of diseases. The process of producing enhanced chelation of minerals are used in some manufacturing processes of coral calcium and these coral minerals have been reported by Dr. Halstead to be more effective in clinical terms. Marine coral has a greater percentage composition of chelated minerals than fossilized coral, which is another reason to prefer the freshly harvested coral from the ocean.

Many commercial companies have promoted coral calcium from Okinawa as though it is all the same material. However, the harvesting of marine bed coral calcium is much more difficult and costly than merely collecting fossilized coral from beach mines. This fossilized coral has undergone thousands, if not millions, of years of erosion, losing most of its magnesium content and much of its trace metal nutrient content. Also, because of the hype generated by coral calcium testimonials, ***numerous, unscrupulous entre-preneurs are harvesting coral from other locations around the world*** (this coral does not have the desired marine microbes), but lying to their customers and telling them that it comes from Okinawa. Some even go so far as to blend their coral with Okinawan coral so that they can make the claim that it comes from Okinawa. Many, even illegally put the Barefoot name on their bottles.

Therefore, interested consumers of food grade coral must be aware of *"cheap"* coral products sold as food supplements. Some of these cheaper products are not only fossilized coral, but they are coral that is *"cut"* with chalk or other inexpensive forms of inorganic minerals. Therefore, the consumer must be aware of the raw material harvesting of coral in the product that they use. Whilst I support the use of Okinawan coral for health, ***it is a fact that marine based coral has far greater health-giving potential than fossilized coral.***

Fortunately, the FDA does do some things correctly as it forces the manufacturers of nutrient products to put the ingredients on the label. It is therefore very simple to tell which product is authentic as marine coral has 12% magnesium in the coral and 25% calcium. The knock off products, which are usually very pricey, will have less than 1% magnesium from the coral, although many times magnesium is added (in which case it will not be from the coral) and the calcium content will be about 35%. Therefore, a glance at the label is all it takes to protect yourself.

The vast majority of allopathic treatments, (drugs and surgery) that are the mainstay of Western Medicine, kill. *Hundreds of thousands die in hospitals every year.* On the other hand, God's nutrients have never been proven to kill any one. God's nutrients, like vitamin-D and its biological partner calcium, cure. Coral calcium has the distinct advent-age of being compatible with many other therapies, and no one has ever reported an allergic reaction to coral. And it has helped many people providing a wholesome mineral support for many body functions. *Coral calcium has a 600 year documented history, in conjunction with the people of Okinawa being out in the sun all day long producing large quantities of vitamin-D*. Millions All over the world have benefited. No other natural nutrient combination has such a track record.

After many years of personal research, we have been able to explain many, although not all, of the reasons for its health giving potential. Coral calcium is begging to be studied in controlled clinical trials. This is the mandate of the FDA, which refuses to do so because coral is a natural sub-stance, food, and therefore cannot be patented for drug industry profit. The tragedy is that the FDA rarely examines any of the tens of thousands of scientific claims made on food substances, such as calcium, by the world's best scientists. *The FDA should take the word "food" out of their name, as they have proven from their track record that they have no right to use it.* What makes this all a big crime is that coral calcium along with its biological partner, vitamin-D will one day, without doubt and without FDA approval, *"cure the world"*:.

But first, let's start in America, start with our friends, start with the Black community. Let's cure the kids and give them a real future instead of the pain and death that now awaits them. Marine grade coral calcium along with vitamin-D supplementation accompanied by a lifestyle change that includes sunshine is all that is needed to prolong your life and be healthy to the end. I am begging all of my Black friends to please follow the Barefoot protocol and maybe live to 100.

I believe it is important to end this book the way it began, and that is to re-emphasis the racial discrimination by the FDA, FTC and AMA against the Black American community. Thus I will repeat a paragraph from chapter one.

In my life, I have never seen a worse form of racial prejudice. Millions of Blacks have died prematurely, in pain and needlessly. If white Americans were dying six years before the Blacks and if they had twice the disease, the regulatory authorities would be spending hundreds of billions of dollars to find out why. These same agencies, the FDA, the FTC and the AMA have not spent one dime to date on the Blacks. Why??? The only reasonable answer is racial prejudice. Because of my passion on this subject, many in the Black American community have tried to get Oprah Winfrey to talk to me, but unfortunately, she has a wall of protection around her that decides for her what she should hear. If she would one day be able to listen, my message to her would be, *"Let's cure humanity, starting with Black America a first."*

Join Bob Barefoot. Let's cure America, let's cure Canada, let's cure our kids and let's cure all humanity. Only then can we cure the world and take the needless pain and degradation out of death

Recommendation by United States Congressman, Howard W. Pollock

The best remedy for the medical disaster looming over America would be an *amendment to the American Constitution enshrining medical freedom*; thereby, allowing both doctors and patients the right to practice and to preach preventive medicine: However, amendments to the Constitution are very rare, and require years to succeed. The American public is desperate today, and cannot wait for this urgently needed change. Thus the best interim remedy would be for each state and the U.S. Congress to legislate an *Alternative Medicine Protection Act* to read as follows:

(**Howard W. Pollock**, Former Territorial Chairman of the Legislative Committee on Statehood for Alaska, and First Republican U.S. Congressman for Alaska.)

"A practitioner of traditional or alternative medicine, registered by an appropriate government authority, who engages in medical or nutritional therapy or in any relevant health procedure, including the recommendation or sale of health supplements, that departs from orthodox or conventional medical

treatment, shall not be found to be unqualified, unprofessional, negligent nor guilty of assault upon a patient, nor be denied the right to pursue her or his professional practice or livelihood, solely on the basis that the therapy employed is an alternative remedy, or is non traditional or departs prevailing orthodox medical treatment, unless it can be conclusively demonstrated that the therapy has a safety risk for a particular patient unreasonably greater than the traditional or prevailing treatment usually employed for the patient's ailment."